Managing Healthcare Ethically

SECOND EDITION

AN EXECUTIVE'S GUIDE

Managing Healthcare Ethically

SECOND
EDITION

AN EXECUTIVE'S GUIDE

William A. Nelson
and Paul B. Hofmann, Editors

ACHE Management Series

Your board, staff, or clients may also benefit from this book's insight. For more information on quantity discounts, contact the Health Administration Press Marketing Manager at (312) 424-9470.

15   14   13   12   11   5   4   3   2   1

Library of Congress Cataloging-in-Publication Data

Managing healthcare ethically / William A. Nelson, Paul B. Hofmann. — 2nd ed.
    p. cm.
  ISBN 978-1-56793-344-4
  1. Health services administration—Moral and ethical aspects. I. Nelson, Bill (William A.)
II. Hofmann, Paul B., 1941-
  RA971.M34635 2009
  362.1068—dc22
                        2009027742

The paper used in this publication meets the minimum requirements of American National Standard for Information Sciences—Permanence of Paper for Printed Library Materials, ANSI Z39.48-1984. ⊚™

Found an error or a typo? We want to know! Please e-mail it to hap1@ache.org, and put "Book Error" in the subject line.

Acquisitions editor: Janet Davis; Project manager: Dojna Shearer; Book designer: Scott Miller; Cover designer: Deb Tremper

Health Administration Press
A division of the Foundation of the
    American College of Healthcare Executives
1 North Franklin Street, Suite 1700
Chicago, IL 60606-3529
(312) 424-2800

To healthcare executives who, by managing ethically, have demonstrated a commitment to improving patient care quality, creating a just culture, and maximizing community benefit

Contents

Foreword

SINCE ITS INCEPTION in 1933, the American College of Healthcare Executives has made ethics and ethical behavior a pillar of the organization. It remains so today; in fact, one of ACHE's four core values is integrity: "We advocate and emulate high ethical conduct in all we do."

Upholding this ideal begins with ACHE's *Code of Ethics*, which was established in 1941. While we rigorously enforce the code, we realize that a reactive approach is not enough on its own. That is why we have also taken proactive approaches to upholding the ethics of the profession, such as

- our many Ethical Policy Statements (see Part V of this book), which are designed to guide ethical decision making;
- the Ethics Self-Assessment (included on page 296), which helps healthcare executives determine areas in which they are on strong ethical ground and areas in which they may need improvement;
- ACHE's annual ethics seminar at the Congress on Healthcare Leadership;
- the annual ethics program that is funded in part by ACHE's philanthropic initiative, the Fund for Innovation in Healthcare Leadership; and

- the Ethics Toolkit, residing on **ache.org**, which provides guidance for understanding and applying the *Code of Ethics,* policy statements, self-assessment, and other ethics resources.

The Healthcare Management Ethics column in *Healthcare Executive* magazine, which has been a part of the magazine since 1992, has been a major contribution to the field and to our affiliates. ACHE is especially pleased to publish this second edition of *Managing Healthcare Ethically: An Executive's Guide,* edited by William A. Nelson, MDiv, PhD, and Paul B. Hofmann, DrPH, FACHE, who are regular contributors to the column. Drs. Nelson and Hofmann are recognized experts in healthcare management ethics and real leaders in our field. They have helped ACHE and its affiliates address ethical issues in countless ways.

I want to take this opportunity to thank them for their many contributions. I also want to thank the other authors who have contributed to *Healthcare Executive* and this publication for their wisdom and their passion for upholding ethics in healthcare management.

The American College of Healthcare Executives is proud of its contributions to the field of healthcare management ethics. This publication is one more step on this ongoing quest.

Thomas C. Dolan, PhD, FACHE, CAE
President and Chief Executive Officer
American College of Healthcare Executives

Acknowledgments

WE WANT TO express our appreciation to the many authors who contributed to the book. Without their effort, neither this book nor *Healthcare Executive*'s Healthcare Management Ethics column would exist. In addition, we would like to acknowledge the editors of *Healthcare Executive* for their wisdom in promoting such a regular feature in ACHE's magazine. We also want to thank Janet Davis and her colleagues at Health Administration Press for quickly accepting our recommendation to publish this second edition, and Dojna Shearer for her editing assistance. Furthermore, we want to thank the many healthcare executives and managers who have attended ACHE's ethics education programs. Each participant has contributed to our growth by raising questions and sharing experiences. We also want to acknowledge and thank Tom Dolan and Deborah Bowen for their commitment and unwavering leadership in supporting the essential role of ethics education for healthcare executives.

William A. Nelson
Paul B. Hofmann

Introduction

HEALTHCARE EXECUTIVES ENCOUNTER ethical challenges that require a decision or an action every day. Ethical decisions involve making the right choice in the face of competing values and options—determining what decision, action, or behavior is best when there is conflict or uncertainty. Executives and managers often struggle to make the right choice. It's seldom easy. Executives' responses to competing values reflect on their leadership and on the organization. Ethical decision making can be complex and challenging and can present significant personal and organizational ramifications.

Every component of the healthcare delivery system is under intense pressure to acknowledge its deficits and accelerate its improvement efforts. Consequently, healthcare executives are being held more accountable; increased transparency is expected and demanded; access, quality, and cost metrics are routinely compared; and resource allocation decisions are under greater scrutiny. If we can respond creatively, effectively, and ethically in this environment, not only will our institutions, patients, and staff be better served, but so will our communities. Ethics is a central foundation of a high-quality organizational culture.

Not surprisingly, there is no comprehensive ethical cookbook with recipes for addressing every potential conflict. But we can draw selectively from the extensive and expanding organizational and clinical ethics literature for assistance. By capitalizing on the insights of professionals who have dealt with these frequently overlapping areas of clinical and organizational ethics, executives will more successfully anticipate and resolve the challenges they represent.

The overarching goal of this book is simple but daunting: to foster quality care. Achieving quality requires a strong commitment to ethical behavior and leadership, ethics-grounded values and culture, and an effective program that promotes ethical actions and practices and clarifies those practices when needed. We offer this edition as a practical resource and guide in addressing that goal.

This second edition of *Managing Healthcare Ethically* contains more than 60 Healthcare Management Ethics columns from *Healthcare Executive* to guide executives and managers in making personal and organizational decisions. Most of the columns selected for this edition appeared in *Healthcare Executive* after the January/February 2001 issue. Sixteen of the selected columns come from the previous edition of this book. In making the difficult decision about which columns to exclude, we removed those that appeared redundant, less relevant, or too narrowly focused.

The 24 authors' perspectives reflect diverse backgrounds as executives, physicians, scholars, teachers, consultants, and ethicists. These authors share a common interest in promoting the development of ethical leaders and ethical healthcare organizations. In this regard, the language of the Joint Commission is quite unambiguous. The purpose of its organizational ethics standards is to "improve care, treatment, services, and outcomes by recognizing and respecting the rights of each patient and by conducting business in an ethical manner." Implicit in this statement is a firm conviction that the content of an organization's vision, mission, and value statements must be more than mere rhetoric. The daily decisions, actions, and behavior of everyone engaged in its programs and services should reflect the values inherent in these statements.

However, ethical conflicts that push executives beyond conventional thinking about the "right" course of action are inevitable.

Competent, reasonable people—including board members, executives, physicians and other clinicians, managers, nonsupervisory employees, patients, families, public officials, and community members—can and will disagree. One's uncertainty or conflicts can be reconciled by applying the following thoughtful, systematic ethics reflection process.

- Clarify the ethics question or uncertainty and the values in conflict.
- Describe the relevant facts surrounding the ethical uncertainty and determine what additional information is needed.
- Identify and understand the values of the key stakeholders.
- Recognize relevant ethics principles and ethics standards of practice.
- Develop feasible options and review the potential benefits and risks associated with each one.
- Select the optimal solution and provide the ethical rationale for the choice.
- Implement the decision.
- Evaluate whether the decision achieved the expected outcome(s) and identify what lessons were learned that might prevent or minimize similar conflicts in the future.

As we stated in the first edition, ethical reflection brings together the values and perspectives of many voices. These columns encourage such a dialogue. Again, their contents rarely give absolute answers, but they provide a guide for exploring conflicts through systematic ethical reflection. The columns examine ethical issues and conflicts in the everyday lives of executives and their organizations. We want to emphasize the importance of integrating ethics discourse and programs into the organization's culture.

In addition to including many new columns, the second edition focuses on the four ethics domains: ethical leadership issues, organizational and management ethics issues, clinical ethics issues, and ethics committees and programs. This edition also contains an expanded section of ACHE ethics tools and resources, including the revised *Code of Ethics*, several new ethics policy statements, and an updated selected bibliography.

Ethics is not and should not be the sole responsibility of an organization's ethics committee or program. No group or individual should serve exclusively as the institution's conscience. An ethical organization is achieved not only through well-crafted policies and procedures; it is achieved when the leadership and the entire staff realize the necessity of ethical thinking and behavior in their routine and daily activities. These columns address patient care issues and the manner in which executives should treat their staff and relate to the broader community.

This book can be used in a variety of ways. It can be read from cover to cover, providing the reader with insights into a wide range of ethical conflicts. Readers can review a particular section or a specific article that corresponds to a conflict they may be experiencing. This book will foster the self-education of executives and managers seeking to enhance their ethics knowledge and skills. You may want to consider reading the stated ethical conflict or question at the beginning of a particular article and pause to think about how you would respond to the conflict before reading the commentary. Such an approach will help you compare your ethical reasoning with that of the author(s). This book can serve as an education resource for a course, a seminar, or an ethics discussion group. However it is used, thoughtful reflection on the various ethical perspectives will enhance your awareness of ethics issues and competing perspectives and values, and it will provide insight into how executive leaders and organizational policy might respond to the ethical conflict.

PART I:
ORGANIZATIONAL
ETHICS LEADERSHIP

ETHICAL ACTIONS AND decision making are key components of professionalism for healthcare executives. The executive's leadership sets the tone for fostering a culture of ethical integrity in an organization. To ensure an ethical organization, executives must consistently demonstrate the importance of integrating ethics into the life of the organization and provide concrete support for its ethics program. Because of the crucial role healthcare executives play in fostering an ethical organization, this topic is placed at the beginning of the book. Part I includes discussions of ethical challenges executives encounter in their role and responsibilities in leading an ethical organization.

Understanding Your Ethical Responsibilities

Frankie Perry, FACHE (R)

TODAY'S COMPLEX HEALTHCARE environment requires that healthcare executives pay even more attention to corporate and personal ethics standards and take the lead to incorporate ethics into day-to-day activities.

Today's healthcare system is a very complex one that's driven by many forces and weighted down by an infinite number of ethical implications. That means more ethical responsibilities for healthcare executives—responsibilities that require healthcare executives to maintain high corporate and personal ethics. These responsibilities also challenge them to balance legal and ethical parameters, act in the best interests of patients, and uphold the organization's mission, often in the face of limited resources.

How do you deal with an HIV-positive physician working with patients in your organization? What about drug and alcohol testing for your employees? Are you making the right moves to stop improper conduct, mishandling of funds, record tampering, sexual harassment, conflicts of interest? Are you meeting the healthcare needs of your community?

First, healthcare executives need to adopt an attitude that makes ethics part of their ongoing decision making and works to build a stronger, more ethically responsive healthcare system. Next, healthcare executives must take a hard look at the way they live and the way they conduct business. Part of that regimen must include an established, practical guide such as the College's *Code of Ethics*, which embraces a professional lifestyle that embodies service, integrity, and leadership.

According to the code, healthcare executives have ethical obligations not only to the healthcare profession, but to society and community as well. These obligations also extend to the organization, the employees, the patients, and those served. It recognizes healthcare executives as the "moral agents" and business conscience of healthcare and requires them to be committed to creating "a more equitable, accessible, effective, and efficient healthcare system." When you join the College, you agree to abide by its Code of Ethics. It's your responsibility to understand this code, honor it, and to report or correct any violations. Actions of affiliates named in violation of the code are evaluated by a grievance procedure enforced by the College's Committee on Ethics. This includes reviewing and investigating cases and then recommending actions to the Board of Governors on allegations brought forth regarding code violations.

The College's Committee on Ethics annually reviews the College's code to make any necessary recommendations regarding updates. In addition, the committee annually issues ethical policy statements to outline current issues and establish recommendations that healthcare executives can use.

The College's *Code of Ethics* and grievance procedures are included in the College's *Annual Report* and *Reference Guide*, which each affiliate receives by mail in November of each year. If you don't have a copy, call [ACHE] for one. If you have not read the code lately, please take a few minutes to do so. In addition, seek out and discuss current articles, books, conferences, and seminars about ethics with your colleagues and management team.

During the months ahead, we hope to strengthen and build the profession's awareness about managerial ethics. The place to start is at the ethical backbone of the healthcare management profession—

the College's *Code of Ethics*. Remember, you represent the College's code. You are the example that everyone in your organization should emulate.

January/February 1992

Can a Manager Be a Moral Leader?

John R. Griffith, FACHE

ANY COMMUNITY DESERVES morally excellent healthcare, and any healthcare organization can be morally improved.

Managers have two tools for promoting moral virtue in their organizations: by example and by using the pragmatic systems of the modern organization to promote moral ends. These mechanisms are not perfect. As to whether they are effective enough to be worth the effort, the answer is that we cannot afford to find out. To be a moral leader, you have to accept the challenge.

PROMOTING VIRTUE BY EXAMPLE

Virtuous managers make moral decisions and show others that it can be done. The more positive examples there are—and the fewer negative ones—the stronger the moral culture of the organization. Recognizing virtuous decisions multiplies the effect of example by the leader. Conversely, a lack of leadership examples and of reward for virtuous decisions destroys a moral culture.

ACTIONS TO PROMOTE MORAL BEHAVIOR

Beyond example, the manager's pragmatic goodness allows the organization to accumulate the resources it needs to make, implement, and reward virtuous decisions. A virtuous organization is almost certainly well-run.

1. Moral leadership is essential, and the higher the rank of the leader the more important the moral character.
2. Sound systems and procedures encourage virtuous acts. Complete and accurate records, internal controls on resources, easy methods to report problems and wrongdoing, rehab programs for substance abuse, and deliberate procedures to protect individual rights all help promote moral virtue.
3. Behavior that is not virtuous must be identified and discouraged. The organization must express this position consistently in its policies, training programs, and operational decisions.
4. Workers should be empowered to the greatest extent possible, and the management style should be participative. Management should establish an environment where difficult issues can be candidly discussed.
5. The organization should offer moral counsel and support, beginning with first-line supervisors. Ethics committees and other resources must be available to support the supervisor and worker.
6. The organization's visible incentives—nonmonetary and monetary—should be based on reward more than blame. Cash rewards and prizes to the worthy may not be necessary if it is clear that they do not accrue to the unworthy.
7. Standard methods of persuasion should be used for moral issues as they are for other human resources concerns. An organization that deliberately promotes morality is likely to get more of it.

8. Leadership should be selected and promoted for moral and non-moral competence. An organization promoting moral virtue pays competitive wages and builds an attractive work environment so it can be selective in recruitment and retention.

Obviously, this is not an easy agenda. Yet any community deserves morally excellent healthcare, and any healthcare organization can be morally improved. Building the momentum meets the moral challenge of healthcare management at its highest level.

May/June 1993

Creating an Organizational Conscience

Paul B. Hofmann, DrPH, FACHE

ACROSS THE COUNTRY, the transformation of the healthcare delivery system is not occurring at the same pace. Eventually, however, every healthcare executive will witness and, in many instances, influence its impact. As this transition proceeds, economic and political pressures will create opportunities for innovative solutions but, at the same time, will produce incentives that can lead to ethical dilemmas for healthcare executives.

Ultimately, it is the CEO's responsibility to establish the moral tone of the organization. A variety of questions can and should be raised to remind each executive that he or she will be held increasingly accountable for both personal and organizational performance from an ethical perspective. Such measurement may be implicit rather than explicit, and yet its importance is undeniable when the moral character of leadership has become suspect in so many fields.

BUILDING TRUST AND CONFIDENCE

How can healthcare executives merit the trust and confidence of their colleagues and the general public? According to the ACHE's

Code of Ethics, executives "must lead lives that embody an exemplary system of values and ethics." No one would argue with this mandate, but what system should be followed?

Familiarity with the classic theories of ethics and values is not required. Instead, as noted by the *Code of Ethics*, the executive is obligated to "conduct all personal and professional activities with honesty, integrity, respect, fairness and good faith." However, unassailable individual behavior is not enough. In view of management's power, authority, and visibility, senior management has the opportunity as well as the obligation to be consistent in their actions and provide vigorous moral leadership.

STAYING ON TRACK

In addition to displaying the virtues that others should emulate, there are two specific actions healthcare executives should consider.

Clarify organizational values

Encourage your board to develop and disseminate a value statement. Too frequently, nonsectarian organizations mistakenly believe this activity is best left to religiously sponsored organizations and serves no purpose for others.

Eventually, every healthcare system, hospital, long-term care facility, home care program, and managed care organization will be forced to make difficult resource allocation decisions involving legitimate alternatives with disparate consequences for their various constituents. When decisions such as these arise, a thorough assessment of organizational values undertaken in an objective fashion and committed to writing can serve as a valuable guide.

Produce and distribute an ethics manual

The ethics manual you produce should contain hypothetical cases depicting the broad spectrum of ethical dilemmas that could be encountered by board members, managers, physicians, employees, and volunteers. Vignettes illustrating potential conflicts of interest, possible violations of confidentiality, questionable discriminatory behavior, and comparable problems can provide instructive examples of how your organization's policies and values should be interpreted.

PROMOTE THE PROCESS

Creating and sustaining an organizational conscience is not easy. During a period when the spotlight is on all aspects of healthcare delivery, it is particularly important to promote the process.

As emphasized by ACHE's *Code of Ethics*, healthcare executives have a wide array of obligations to the profession, to patients or others served, to the organization, to employees, to the community, and to society. Although ACHE's *Code of Ethics* describes these obligations in helpful detail, it is up to healthcare executives to put these words into practice and set the organization's moral tone.

November/December 1994

Balancing Professional and Personal Priorities

Paul B. Hofmann, DrPH, FACHE

THE INTRINSIC GOAL is to achieve and maintain an acceptable equilibrium by continually balancing professional and personal needs. As everyone knows, it is not an easy task.

Every conscientious healthcare executive must contend with high expectations—usually self-imposed—that create inevitable pressure to work both harder and smarter. Priorities are constantly being reassessed and shifted to accommodate new and seemingly more important requirements.

Of course, these demands aren't exclusively professional in nature. Personal and family needs invariably compete with job-related priorities for the healthcare executive's time and attention. Mere time often emerges as the healthcare executive's most precious and least available resource.

So what do we do? We compromise. Intuitively, relative costs and benefits are measured, and a choice is made. By rationalizing misjudgments and rarely acknowledging our fallibility, we manage to cope and hope that others understand. But healthcare executives have an ethical responsibility to their organizations, colleagues, and employees to do more than just cope. We must put personal issues into perspective and maintain balance to perform well professionally.

Ethical behavior has been described as obedience to the unenforceable. In addition to personal values, an executive's behavior is driven by conscience, defined by the dictionary as "the inner sense of what is right or wrong in one's conduct or motives, impelling one toward right action." Consequently, there is no universal prescription healthcare executives can follow to prevent mistakes or ensure ethical behavior.

While no universal prescription exists, there are guideposts that healthcare executives can follow. For example, the ACHE's *Code of Ethics*, with which all affiliates are expected to comply, contains standards of ethical behavior for healthcare executives in their professional relationships. As emphasized in the Code's preamble, leaders should "merit the trust, confidence, and respect of healthcare professionals and the general public. To do so, healthcare executives must lead lives that embody an exemplary system of values and ethics." Healthcare executives should periodically review this document.

MAINTAINING BALANCE

When examining the balance between professional and personal priorities, these questions should be addressed:

- Am I eating properly, getting adequate rest and sufficient exercise, setting realistic expectations, and fostering supportive interpersonal relationships? Vitality, physical as well as mental, is an undeniable prerequisite and ongoing necessity to sustain an appropriate balance.
- Am I sensitive to emotional as well as physical warning signs of imbalance—not only in myself but in others? Am I willing to seek assistance? Healthcare organizations should provide access to counseling and other services to assist staff in addressing problems that adversely affect job performance.
- Do I resolve conflicts quickly? Honesty, commitment, trust,

understanding, and accommodation are among the many attributes required to achieve timely conflict resolution.

Historically, leaders have been more likely to monitor the behavior of subordinates and to intervene when necessary. Perhaps due to executives' perfectionist tendencies, frenetic schedules, and high energy, they are oblivious to the masochistic consequences of their behavior. Unless executives consciously and regularly examine the personal and organizational costs, along with the benefits, of professional achievement, a safe and satisfying balance will not be maintained.

May/June 1994

The Ethics of Downsizing

Paul B. Hofmann, DrPH, FACHE

Your organization has taken every possible step to become more cost-effective, but expenses must be reduced further, and it has become clear a significant number of positions will have to be eliminated. You have been designated as the management person responsible for designing the downsizing plan. How can your plan demonstrate genuine sensitivity to the ethical dimensions of this often painful process?

When addressing this question, healthcare executives should first ask themselves, "What are my organization's objectives for downsizing and how can I measure my success in meeting them?"

Too often, a layoff plan has as its sole objective a reduction in workforce within a designated time frame to decrease salary and benefit costs. Frequently, department heads are requested to submit their proposals for meeting the designated figure, and the human resource director is held accountable for working with other senior executives to ensure appropriate coordination and implementation of these proposals after final approval by the CEO.

While it is important to determine specific downsizing targets, it is also necessary to develop additional objectives for the action. Following are five you might consider adopting as well as appropriate measurement tools:

1. No diminution in quality of patient care.
   - Measurement tool: Results of patient satisfaction question-naires, number and type of incident reports, patient complaints, and changes in other quality indicators.
2. A sustained level of productivity.
   - Measurement tool: Performance, absenteeism, and sick leave reports.
3. Retention of a positive image via focused communication efforts and other programs designed for patients, medical staff, board members, volunteers, and the community.
   - Measurement tool: Number of complaints, tone of media coverage, and other feedback.
4. Effective communication to and support for remaining and departing personnel.
   - Measurement tool: Post layoff survey of current and former employees.
5. A reasonable severance package, including appropriate length of severance payment and continuation of individual benefits (e.g., life insurance, disability insurance, medical benefits), provision of outplacement services, retraining support, and assistance with financial and/or retirement planning.
   - Measurement tool: Number of complaints, formal grievances, and wrongful discharge claims.

In a downsizing effort, management must not be morally neutral. Perhaps the most practical advice I can give is to capitalize on the past experiences of organizations that have dealt with this challenge. A particularly impressive report is "Hospital Layoffs: One Facility's Experience with a Work Force Reduction," by John D. Rudnick, Jr., FACHE, which was published in the September/October 1995 issue of *Health Progress*.

Also, to mitigate the anxiety and distress associated with downsizing measures, healthcare executives can employ a variety of formal actions that are described in the ACHE's Ethical Policy Statement, "Ethical Issues Related to a Reduction in Force" on page 279.

Because almost every healthcare organization will have to reduce payroll costs, if it has not already done so, executives should review this policy statement carefully.

Employees deserve to be treated with fairness and integrity; therefore, executives should not use euphemisms to create insupportable illusions that everyone's needs will be met. Executives may want to refer to "restructuring" and "rightsizing," but these terms are transparent and ominous to the average employee. Feelings of apprehension, fear, and anger usually cannot be entirely eliminated; however, they can be at least partially alleviated by timely, consistent, and honest communication.

November/December 1995

Abuse of Power

Paul B. Hofmann, DrPH, FACHE

As a hospital executive, I am dismayed when I see certain physicians and managers using their power to intimidate patients, families, and staff. What can I do to stop this unethical behavior and prevent it in the future?

Unfortunately, abuse of power is at least as prevalent, if not more so, in healthcare organizations as it is in other types of organizations. Furthermore, because potential consequences are far more severe than in other settings, abuse of power in a clinical facility is particularly objectionable and unacceptable.

Patients and their families are exceptionally vulnerable in a time of crisis. They are apprehensive, sometimes frightened, and often intimidated by the organization's sheer physical size and bureaucratic complexity. Physicians, still at the top of the power structure in many hospitals, generally have a great deal of formal and informal organizational and personal leverage. Therefore, some individuals in authority (physicians as well as other clinical staff) may speak and act inappropriately, but this behavior is tolerated because patients and families often feel too overwhelmed and powerless to voice their objections.

Similar problems occur when managers who have significant authority do not use it for the good of the organization and those it serves. Employees under their supervision can be compromised by their misuse of power, adversely affecting both morale and productivity. Like patients and their families, employees may feel helpless and hesitant to object to such behavior.

Examples of abuse of power include rudeness, profane language, promise breaking, deception, dishonesty, and sexual harassment. Less obvious forms of abuse of power tend to be subtle and therefore more insidious; these include arrogance, use of overly confusing jargon, and withholding of information.

Management and medical staff sometimes rationalize this sort of unprofessional conduct because they view it as unintentional and non-malicious. However, in addition to compromising its immediate victims, tolerating such behavior has several negative long-term consequences, such as encouraging the individual to continue this conduct, silently condoning the behavior and suggesting to others that they can behave in a similar manner with impunity, demoralizing those who become aware of the organization's tolerance, and adversely affecting the image and reputation of the organization.

A variety of action steps can be taken to mitigate the abuse of power. Among them are the following:

- Recognize the inadequacy of well-intentioned rhetoric, including organizational values statements unaccompanied by explicit programs to reinforce them.
- Develop and implement a code of conduct for management, staff, and physicians.
- Perform periodic ethics audits that include questions about abuse of power (see "Performing an Ethics Audit" in the November/December 1995 issue of *Healthcare Executive*).
- Prepare a casebook with descriptions of unacceptable behavior and constructive interventions and use it in management orientation and training sessions.
- Conduct educational programs to promote candid discussion of these issues.

- Establish and encourage the use of a "hotline" to report inappropriate conduct.
- Sanction improper behavior promptly.
- Encourage the referral of physician problems to the medical staff's physician advisory committee.
- Emphasize the importance of sensitivity to the values of patients, families, and staff in routine employee performance appraisals.

Regrettably, it is unlikely that you can totally prevent abuse of power, but constant vigilance and effective intervention can reduce its incidence. Most importantly, you cannot achieve this objective unless senior management and clinical leaders themselves demonstrate zero tolerance for insensitive and inappropriate behavior.

March/April 1999

Allocating Limited Capital Resources

Paul B. Hofmann, DrPH, FACHE

Predictably, we always receive more project requests than can be accommodated by our capital budget. In addition to the traditional financial criteria, are there ethical factors that should be considered when a choice must be made among equally compelling requests?

Invariably, healthcare executives are asked to approve capital expenditures in excess of available funds. And given the unrelenting economic pressures to provide more services with less reimbursement, this situation will not abate in the near future.

CONVENTIONAL APPROACH

Historically, decision makers have relied almost exclusively on well-tested criteria to assess the impact of a proposed project or piece of equipment. Among them are

- meeting the needs of various constituencies (patients, physicians, employees, and others);
- improving the cost-effectiveness of service (including safety, length of stay, access, and productivity);

- complying with legal, licensing, regulatory, and Joint Commission requirements; and
- satisfying financial viability measures (time period to obtain return on investment, contribution margin per case, probability of achieving forecast).

The use of these and similar evaluation criteria to make an objective, sound decision is both appropriate and essential, but not sufficient. This is especially true when you are confronted with proposals that appear equally compelling. A comprehensive cost-benefit comparison should be complemented by an ethical analysis. The ultimate goal, of course, is to make decisions that are not only economically justified but also morally defensible.

APPLICATION OF ETHICAL PRINCIPLES

A review of the literature on ethics and ethical theory suggests that a wide range of ethical principles could be relevant to the capital budget decision-making process; however, the following four have specific relevance.

- **Beneficence** could be defined as acting with charity and kindness, but this definition is inadequate. Fully embracing the principle requires actively promoting behaviors that benefit others. The key term here is "active"; passivity fundamentally violates the basic integrity of the concept. With many nonprofit hospitals vulnerable to allegations that they do not provide sufficient community benefit to justify their tax-exempt status, the ability of some organizations to literally document their beneficence may influence long-term organizational survival.
- **Nonmaleficence** prohibits doing harm to others. A healthcare executive has an indisputable obligation to take no action that would injure the organization or those it serves. For example, by avoiding misconduct that could result in compromising the

organization and its staff, management refuses to engage in activities that might represent a conflict of interest. This is not simply a hypothetical concern. Capital expenditure decisions could easily be made that may have personal and/or institutional value to the detriment of the community, such as supporting a project advocated by a board member rather than funding an indigent care clinic.

- **Fidelity** suggests adherence to a contract or covenant to fulfill certain responsibilities. This principle also connotes fulfilling one's duty and keeping promises. In the context of deciding among competing proposals, all of them being highly desirable, which one will be most supportive of the organization's overall mission and values? A thoughtful, dispassionate examination of each proposal's relevance to sustaining the current and future mission should be an indispensable part of the analysis. Similarly, if a request is not aligned with your organization's values, it should compare unfavorably with competing applications for capital funds.

- **Justice** implies a responsibility to act with fairness and impartiality. Although it is difficult to argue that any of the principles should "trump" another, an appropriate resource allocation decision cannot be made unless it is fair and impartial. Not only should the distribution of resources reflect fairness, but the outcome should also consider the legacy of previous inequities. Consequently, justice mandates a complete exploration of the moral traces resulting from past practices of discrimination, as well as activities that were influenced by different circumstances and priorities. Earlier appropriation decisions could have been affected by political factors that are no longer applicable. These past actions must be taken into consideration when making resource allocation decisions today.

Healthcare executives, like those in other fields, practice the fine art of the possible, becoming ever more proficient in making organizational compromises by negotiating politically acceptable solutions. Determining which capital proposals will be approved when all cannot be funded, regardless of their sound justification, often requires a delicate balancing process. The more thorough and comprehensive the assessment, incorporating both economic and noneconomic criteria, the more likely the outcome will be both prudent and just.

March/April 2000

Coping with Staffing Shortages

Benn J. Greenspan, PhD, FACHE

My organization has a range of acute clinical services that are often used to physical capacity. Because our region is experiencing broad labor shortages, staffing levels are not always what we would like or need them to be, which presents us with the dilemma of whether to continue to accept patients. What are our ethical obligations?

As it becomes increasingly difficult to fill nursing, ancillary, and other related positions, healthcare providers must be clear about the standards and objectives used to protect patients, staff, and the integrity of their organizations. While a fundamental objective of healthcare management is to ensure the well-being of patients, we must also pursue equitable, accessible, effective, and efficient provision of healthcare. Even in the best of circumstances, the simultaneous pursuit of efficacy and efficiency may require compromise between these two goals—and may also create inherent conflicts that are exacerbated when resources are limited.

In raising your question, you already recognize the conflict between the level of service you want to provide and the service that is possible with your limited resources. How can you resolve this conflict?

Triage, or rationing, is an intrinsic method of providing healthcare.

Regardless of staffing levels, healthcare providers must always allocate limited resources. For example, not every patient receives one-to-one nursing care, and not every patient recovers in a bed with an automated system to minimize skin pressure. Patients are supposed to receive the care they need. When resources are limited, these decisions can be more difficult; however, it is never a question of whether we will do what is necessary, only how we will do it.

As healthcare executives, we often rely on our organizations' missions for guidance when we face such ethical dilemmas. Formulating specific guidelines in advance of staffing shortages will help your organization choose the "right" response to a real-life situation in which there is no single response—only several answers that may conflict. Taking the following actions will help you create effective policies and procedures.

Define levels of service. Openly establish a suitable understanding of what (apart from the "desired" levels of professional service) are the minimum acceptable and appropriate standard levels of service that will not compromise patient well-being. Be clear that while your organization may of course exceed the minimum acceptable standard, it must commit to never dropping below it. These levels must also be based on existing standards that have been promulgated through statute, regulation, and accreditation guidelines.

Achieve organizational consensus. Be sure that standard service levels are agreed upon with input from your staff and board. Achieving consensus through open discussion of these standards is necessary in order to

- ensure that the well-being of patients is not eclipsed by the stresses of staffing shortages,
- assure your staff that they are not being asked to offer care that is below the standards of what is expected by the profession at large,
- assure your board that your organization has exercised due process in the pursuit of standards of care,
- let all members of your community know that you are committed

to optimizing your ability to deliver the best care possible, and

- satisfy your community's needs for high-quality service.

Create a reporting mechanism. Your organization must establish a mechanism through which staff can express concern when they believe that the minimum service level is being approached. As a result of using this resource, staff should expect that effective, reasonable action will be taken. The mechanism must be open, legitimate, objective, responsive, and nonretributive.

If you receive reports of subpar service, you can take one of the following actions:

- If you are a sole community provider, perform classic triage to determine who can be safely sent home.
- Shorten the length of stay for some patients. This measure can relieve resource pressure, improve organizational efficiency, and encourage alternatives—such as home care—that often improve patient satisfaction.
- Develop resource-sharing agreements with other organizations.
- In departments that are overloaded, refer patients to neighboring providers.

If the options listed are not available, you may have to take the ultimate step of refusing to provide elective patient care until the crisis period has passed. This decision might be necessary to safeguard patients, to recognize the ethical mandates of staff, and to preserve the integrity of your organization.

In following this process, we are recognizing the critical principle of nonmaleficence—attempting to minimize the potential to do harm to each patient—and its balance with the principles of beneficence and justice—alleviating the suffering of others to the broadest degree possible. By making the process open and inclusive, we are acknowledging the professional and ethical demands on our staff to pursue fidelity and honesty in serving our patients. We also maximize and benefit from the creative abilities of staff, board members, and our community in finding better ways to address important problems—a strategy that can prove invaluable in the face of an uncertain future.

May/June 2001

The Values of a Profession

Everett A. Johnson, PhD, LFACHE

IN EVERY PROFESSION, a set of values—be it formal or informal—guides the behavior of individuals as they carry out their primary duties. For example, the chief financial officer of a business is responsible for maintaining a financially solvent organization within an ethical context; in medicine, clinicians take an oath to "do no harm" to the patient.

Those who choose a career in healthcare management are in the unique position of committing themselves to the values of business and medicine. At their core, both professions are guided by a similar quest to deliver the highest quality care possible. Yet as the needs of today's healthcare organizations often exceed available resources, administrative and medical concerns may occasionally seem to conflict with one another.

Balancing administrative and medical values can become a serious dilemma for healthcare executives when difficult decisions must be made. This challenge may be further complicated by the competing expectations of the other constituents that a healthcare organization serves. In addition to the needs of physicians and patients that should be considered, the business community, government agencies, and social service organizations may also express varying—and at times, conflicting—expectations. In situations where decisions are viewed by different constituencies as a choice between values, how should healthcare executives proceed?

Perhaps the best way executives can address such situations is to examine their leadership style and the system of values that their style sets for the organization. Effective leaders create an environment in which the values of the organization and the field of healthcare management are clear. Thus, when executives are faced with decisions that the organization's key stakeholders view as a choice between values, the course of action will be judged as fair. Following are several ways healthcare executives can foster an environment that embodies the values of healthcare management.

- **Place trust in the decision-making abilities of staff.** The freedom to make decisions without fear of reprisal is a necessary characteristic for superior performance. Excellent patient care occurs when caregivers are free to make professional decisions. Healthcare executives have a duty to encourage creativity and develop decision-making skills among staff at all levels of the organization. This creates respect and encourages collaboration between leadership and staff as well as administrators and clinicians.
- **Take accountability for subordinates.** In large organizations with several hierarchical levels, staff may make decisions that senior-level leaders are unaware of for quite some time. When employees fail to make appropriate decisions, the responsibility for those actions ultimately falls upon the organization's leadership. To blame an associate and deny responsibility creates distrust throughout the organization.
- **Be visible to caregivers on a daily basis.** Letting a hectic schedule justify administering from one's office is shortsighted. Executives who do so must then rely on internal reporting systems to bring problems to the forefront. Because minor issues that are easily ignored can later become major problems, executives who are visible and available on an informal basis have an opportunity to sense their staff's problems and to address those problems in a compassionate and timely manner.

- **Help staff gain perspective.** When hard choices must be faced, the healthcare organization's constituents need to understand how their opinions, values, and expectations affect the organization as a whole. To facilitate understanding, executives can place conflicts in a wider perspective by being objective and forthright in addressing issues and sharing information. On major issues, timidity to initiate discussion may cause confusion and decrease confidence in the organization's leaders.
- **Lead with a consistent style and focus.** Senior-level leaders must be predictable in their decision making and actions. Uncertainty will lead to distrust and possibly diminish staff performance.

Effective leadership also requires healthcare executives to think about the emotional needs of constituents and to respond with both concern and caring that mirrors these feelings. In weighing the outcomes of a decision, consider the following questions:

- Does the decision demonstrate an appreciation for patients and staff?
- Does it conform to acceptable conduct?
- Does it show solicitude and the ideals of caring?
- Does it demonstrate careful attention to the implications of the decision?
- Is it consistent with and does it reinforce the vision and mission of the organization?

The values demonstrated through an executive's leadership style send a clear signal—both internally and to the community—of the values held by the organization. When leaders strive to pursue excellence in a just and fair manner, the entire organization will be inspired to reach for outstanding performance.

March/April 2002

Why Good People Behave Badly

Paul B. Hofmann, DrPH, FACHE

Having worked in several different organizations, I have noticed otherwise good people behaving poorly under different circumstances. What accounts for this variability and what can be done about it?

Michael Daignault, formerly of the Ethics Resource Center in Washington, DC, once described why good people do bad things. He cited a long list of generic reasons, but the following are particularly relevant in today's healthcare environment.

- **They do not feel loyal to the organization.** Predictably, this occurs most often among short-term employees and in organizations with high staff turnover.
- **They feel pressure to "succeed" as defined by the organization.** For example, those organizations placing greater emphasis on net income than on clinical outcome, and valuing conformity over candor, are more likely to have personnel who act inappropriately and unethically. Fraud and abuse violations by a number of national healthcare systems and prominent medical centers were undoubtedly motivated, at least in part, by an overemphasis on financial criteria.
- **They feel entitled.** An inflated sense of self-importance and

an absence of organizational pride usually contribute to a feeling of entitlement.

- **They believe that the rules do not apply to them.** Just as some people drive over the speed limit, rationalizing that their business is more urgent and they are better drivers than others, there are employees who will assert that they should not be subject to certain policies and procedures.
- **They do not view the act as illegal.** Despite the common perception that an act is ethical if it's legal, the law is usually a minimum standard. In a 1994 *Harvard Business Review* article, "Managing for Organizational Integrity," Lynn Sharp Paine wrote, "Managers who define ethics as legal compliance are implicitly endorsing a code of moral mediocrity for their organizations."
- **They feel pressured by their peers.** This influence naturally begins in early childhood and usually extends consciously or unconsciously throughout one's personal and professional life.
- **They lack resources.** "Cutting corners" to save time or dollars is a convenient excuse for doing something that most people would agree is wrong when resources are plentiful.

Belatedly, there is growing recognition of another pervasive element, indeed an insidious factor, contributing to the failure of good people to do the right thing: bad systems. It may be a truism that a poorly designed, ineffective system will trump a well-intentioned person almost every time. David M. Messick and Max H. Bazerman, in a 1996 *Sloan Management Review* article, "Ethical Leadership and Psychology of Decision Making," noted when an employee acts badly, we tend to contrast him or her with better workers, rather than ask if there is something encouraging bad behavior. If compounded by inconsistent policies and marginally effective computer systems, defective processes can and do complicate the ability of good people to do the right thing.

Actually, when resources are adequate, when controversy is absent, when there is no sense of great urgency, when there are no conflicts of interest and when neither ambiguity nor ambivalence exists, decisions may still be hard, but acting ethically when merely convenient is hardly acceptable. It is precisely during times of limited resources, conflicting opinions, severe time constraints, competing loyalties, significant uncertainty, and potential personal risk that good people are most likely to make and rationalize bad decisions. Unfortunately, denial and rationalization have become useful forms of ethical amnesia.

The relevance of an organization's vision, mission, and values statements should not be minimized in promoting high standards of personal conduct. Similarly, having an ethics officer, code of ethics, sound policies, and comprehensive training programs are all important, but they are not sufficient. Enron had all of these.

Ultimately, as is the case so often, a comprehensive program fostering ethical behavior will succeed or fail based upon the example established by one person: the CEO. If he or she follows Carson Dye's admonitions to adopt a personal code of ethics, to weigh the cost of not being ethical, to tell the truth and not exaggerate, to ensure that actions match words, to use power appropriately, and to admit mistakes (*Leadership in Healthcare: Values at the Top*), then the inclination of good people to do bad things will be much less.

Past experience, however, should remind us of one caveat. Strong leaders can inspire vision, creativity, trust, passion, and pride, but these are not enough. Unless accompanied by the attributes of competency, transparency, integrity, and humility, good people could still emulate a leader lacking a solid ethical compass.

The final litmus test is when staff members, regardless of their organizational status, do not hesitate in choosing the hard right over the easy wrong.

March/April 2004

Addressing Rural Ethics Issues

William A. Nelson, PhD

I have recently accepted a position as the CEO of a small, rural health-care organization. In my previous position as vice president of operations at an urban facility, I actively served on the organization's ethics committee. What are the different ethical challenges I might face serving on an ethics committee in a rural setting?

Since rural facilities are less likely to have ethics committees than their urban counterparts, it is notable that your organization has such an important resource. Just like urban ethics committees, rural committees vary in functions, sophistication, leadership, and respect. In both settings, committee members must apply ethical principles and standards to site-specific conflicts or questions. Rural ethics are distinct in terms of the conflicts that occur, not the principles or standards used to address them.

Despite the extent of published analysis on a variety of ethical conflicts, little has been written specifically about rural healthcare ethics. Although it is difficult to generalize about a particular geographical area, growing evidence supports the claim that unique ethical issues arise in a rural healthcare setting.

Many challenges relate to the general geographical and social characteristics of the delivery of healthcare in a rural setting. Some characteristics that raise ethical questions include:

- **Homogeneous values and cultural perspective.** Racial and ethnic diversity has spread beyond the city; however, rural communities continue to share common values, such as self-reliance and independence, and cultural perspectives that influence healthcare practices in their regions.
- **Limited economic resources.** Rural healthcare organizations encounter distinct economic challenges. For example, the number of patients living below the poverty level is higher than in most major metropolitan areas, while the per capita income is lower.
- **Rural population health status.** Statistically, rural populations tend to become sick more often and are typically older, with higher death rates than urban populations.
- **Limited access to care.** Across the country, many rural counties have limited access to—or simply nonexistent—healthcare organizations or healthcare professionals, including nurses, social workers, and mental health professionals.
- **Fewer specialized healthcare providers.** Rural physicians tend to be family practitioners, in contrast with urban settings in which a wide variety of specialized care providers are readily available.
- **Distance between healthcare professionals.** In rural areas, the distance to and between healthcare professionals and facilities can be extensive. Furthermore, reaching large medical centers, especially in crisis moments, can be extremely difficult.
- **Dual and overlapping relationships between a healthcare professional's work life and personal life.** In smaller communities, the buffer between the provider or administrator and patient can be small. When "everyone" knows the provider or administrator, regular contact can occur with the patient almost anywhere at any time.

Ethical issues faced in the rural healthcare setting are significantly influenced by these general characteristics. Aside from the commonly recognized ethical issues, such as end-of-life decision making, following are several of the most common clinical and organizational ethical issues that your rural ethics committee will routinely address:

- Confidentiality and privacy
- Boundary and multirelationship issues
- Referral and transfer issues
- Allocation of limited resources both locally and nationally
- Shared decision-making issues
- Conflict of interest
- Quality of care

As in any setting, the process for responding involves the systematic application of ethical standards or principles to the particular conflict. For example, issues related to confidentiality can be uniquely challenging in a rural setting, where people live in such close proximity that they have frequent contact with members of the community. Complicating the issue may be the community culture that encourages openness and sharing. A vice president of a small hospital could regularly encounter a friend at a gathering or local store and be asked, "I hear our neighbor is at the hospital. How is he doing?"

Ethical conflicts regarding confidentiality should be anticipated by the ethics committee and those in leadership positions. Since many of these rural ethics issues are of a recurring nature, the ethics committee—in consultation with healthcare executives—should proactively explore such conflicts by reviewing the ethics literature, professional guidelines, and consensus documents to develop local ethical standards of practice. By prospectively recognizing the ethical challenges and developing ethical standards of practice, the organization can prevent significant conflicts from occurring, as well as have guidelines prepared for all staff when situations arise. The standards can be propagated by the ethics committee. This process will not eliminate the need for a competent and available ethics consultation program or resource. When needed, the committee's ethics consultation process can clarify the standards of practice.

Therefore, as an experienced ethics committee member, you will be able to apply the same basic ethical standards you used in the urban setting. However, you will need to identify the unique conflicts in your rural setting that require thoughtful, systematic ethical guidance.

July/August 2004

Responsibility for Unsuccessful Promotions

Paul B. Hofmann, DrPH, FACHE

Highly skilled clinical people are frequently promoted to management positions, but many fail to perform successfully in their new role. Is this an ethical issue? If so, how can it be avoided?

Commonly, organizations view promoting an employee as an opportunity to reward excellent work and loyalty. Although well motivated, such an action is clearly not justified if the individual is unqualified to assume supervisory responsibility. People can be attracted by more status and compensation, but if they lack management skills and interest, we unintentionally do them a great disservice by assuming everyone must want to experience the "joys" of an administrative role.

This issue is not simply an ethical matter. Nonetheless, appointing a managerially unskilled person and/or failing to deal with an incompetent supervisor can carry a very significant ethical cost. Inappropriate decisions by such an individual not only may compromise patient care but also can adversely affect subordinates, peers, and the person to whom he or she reports. Therefore, everyone is potentially compromised, including the new supervisor.

The virtues of internal promotions are important to recognize. Every progressive organization should encourage employees to pursue career advancement within their organization. Candidates for entry-level positions are usually attracted to an employer that has a strong record of internal promotions, and current staff members are more likely to remain if they witness tangible evidence of such activity. In addition, promoting an internal applicant is almost always easier, faster, and less costly than appointing someone from outside. Finally, the level of comfort and familiarity with a current employee is usually much higher in comparison with an external applicant.

PREVALENCE OF FALSE ASSUMPTIONS

Several widely held false assumptions help explain why people are often promoted beyond their level of competency.

- A person with good technical or clinical skills is qualified for a supervisory position. Because this employee is an exemplary nurse, pharmacist, physical therapist, social worker, laboratory or X-ray technologist, he or she surely will be an excellent manager.
- Every nonsupervisory employee aspires to have a management position. We have gauged our own success based upon progressing through the administrative ranks, so we believe the same is true of others.
- Individuals are unlikely to be seduced by the allure of higher pay and benefits, a new title, and perhaps an office if they are not genuinely interested in the promotion. Although these factors are important to us, the average person will be able to look objectively at the advantages and disadvantages of the new role.
- Someone invited by a supervisor, department head, or senior executive to apply for a specific opening will be entirely comfortable in declining the invitation. Despite the implicit expectation that the person will be flattered, we cannot imagine that the individual would hesitate to turn down the suggestion if there were any serious reservations.

STEPS TO PREVENT UNWISE APPOINTMENTS

Five steps are recommended to avoid the problems associated with appointing unqualified candidates:

1. Do not underestimate the leadership, planning, financial, and other skills required to perform effectively as a supervisor; make sure that the position description accurately documents the full range of responsibilities.
2. Avoid rationalizing that the time, effort, and cost of external recruitment are not worth the investment, even when viable internal candidates are available; encourage such candidates to apply to facilitate a fair comparison of qualifications.
3. Do not understate the number or magnitude of challenges inherent in the position during the interview process; a full disclosure of these challenges and the organization's expectations permits an informed decision by the successful candidate and reduces the likelihood of subsequent recriminations.
4. Identify employees who have the potential for advancement and an interest in promotional opportunities; encourage them to participate in supervisory development courses and to attend selected seminars and conferences.
5. Provide sufficient financial incentives and status to reward staff with superior skills who do not have an interest in or aptitude for significant administrative responsibility.

Almost every organization has some supervisors who are marginally capable. The managers to whom they report could be reluctant to take disciplinary action because it is personally painful and difficult. Rationalizations abound: The supervisor has been with the organization for a long time, is such a nice person, is close to retirement, is related to an influential member of the medical staff or board of trustees, is the sole income earner for the family, is likely to file a complaint, etc. An effective executive, however, who is administratively competent and ethically sensitive will take steps to minimize the number of such supervisors by creating and sustaining an organizational culture in which only truly qualified candidates are encouraged to be applicants.

January/February 2005

Confronting Management Incompetence

Paul B. Hofmann, DrPH, FACHE

Too many executives do not deal in a timely way with incompetent or marginally competent managers. Why is this an ethics issue and how should it be addressed?

In healthcare, as in every field, one of the most fundamental and challenging responsibilities of a leader is to tackle tough and uncomfortable situations promptly and effectively. If an otherwise very capable executive has only one shortcoming, it will often be the failure to move decisively when a senior officer, department head, or supervisor is performing poorly.

Failing to take action constitutes a grave ethical lapse. Staff morale suffers when incompetence is tolerated and even rewarded. Unfortunately, depending on their area of responsibility, incompetent managers eventually compromise patient care, subordinates, peers, and possibly the organization itself. Furthermore, failing to address this issue harms the executive's moral authority to lead.

Ironically, the ineffectiveness of a particular manager is rarely a secret. Subordinates are certainly aware of the problem, as are peers and others who must contend with this person's inadequate performance. Ineffectual managers themselves are usually aware of their deficiencies, although they may have difficulty admitting the need for improvement.

Remarkably, executives may not fully appreciate that their own position is at risk. If inferior performance is tolerated for an extended period, leadership's credibility inevitably will be adversely affected. Key members of the organization will raise legitimate questions: Does senior management know there is a problem? If it does, why is nothing being done? If an executive does not realize a manager is not performing well, why not?

REASONS FOR PROCRASTINATION

Assuming that performance problems of an ineffective manager are known and irreversible, there are a number of reasons why they may not be addressed in a suitable manner:

1. Confronting this issue is hardly enjoyable; indeed, it is the least pleasant part of management and is not usually covered in either undergraduate or graduate courses.
2. Conceding that you may have made a bad hiring or promotion decision will always be hard.
3. Resolving a management performance predicament can consume a significant amount of time and emotional energy.
4. Maintaining the status quo is easier and avoids the uncertainty associated with changes.
5. Overcoming inertia is especially difficult if the person is well liked, hard working, loyal, and conscientious; supports a large family; is within a few years of retirement; has "political" connections; and/or received consistently acceptable performance reviews from prior supervisors.
6. Hoping the individual will still meet clearly agreed on expectations, despite a previous inability to do so, is an illusion that can be rationalized easily.

When interviewing candidates for a senior executive position, among the questions I routinely asked was, "How many people have you terminated in the past five years, and, if you could do it again, would you have handled those decisions any differently?" Typically, one person would say, "I did not terminate anyone; everybody is salvageable." Another might think for a short period and then reply, "I fired four people, it had to be done, and I wouldn't have changed a thing." Invariably, a third candidate would respond, "I had to discharge three, and it was painfully difficult, but perhaps I waited too long." While extending a job offer obviously was not solely dependent on their answers to these questions, this part of the interview conversation always contributed to a better understanding of the candidate's management style and philosophy.

RECOMMENDATIONS

Among other attributes, managing ethically requires competency, courage, and compassion. Assuming again that every reasonable step has been taken to help the individual improve his or her performance to no avail and another more suitable position is not available, each of these attributes is particularly relevant in dealing successfully with a manager whose performance is unacceptable.

Competency in this context means the executive does not rationalize, procrastinate, or naively underestimate the organizational cost of incompetence. Instead, when there is no doubt action must be taken, a comprehensive plan must be carefully prepared. This plan may include

- consultation with legal counsel, human resources, and key people within the organization;
- reviewing documentation of progressive disciplinary action to assure the individual has been properly counseled and to defend an allegation of wrongful discharge;
- consultation with the board and medical staff leaders;
- verification that contractual obligations will be met and severance benefits are accurately determined;

- consideration of additional benefits, such as assistance with job placement; and
- preparation of internal and possibly external announcements, including designation of an interim manager.

Unquestionably, other issues should be considered, but creating and implementing a detailed plan will maximize the likelihood that the transition will be responsive to the needs of the individual and the organization.

Courage is identified as an essential component because most marginally performing managers remain in their positions, not because their inadequacies are unknown, but because their supervisors lack the mettle to take action. Otherwise capable, these leaders may be apprehensive about the institution's informal power structure, feel overextended, and be concerned about the time and effort associated with recruiting a more qualified replacement. Regrettably, they do a great disservice to their organization when they do not demonstrate the courage of their convictions, forcing others to pay a high price for their own timidity.

The term *compassion* is self-explanatory. However, genuine compassion in coping with the unavoidable discomfort associated with discharging a manager or any employee requires empathy for all the participants. Disbelief, anger, recrimination, bargaining, depression, and a host of other emotional reactions should be anticipated. Dealing with managers who have lied, cheated, violated the organization's policies, or committed some other unacceptable act is relatively easy compared with contending with managers who are simply not capable of performing their job despite extensive continuing education, counseling, and other interventions.

Compassion is an important ingredient in a supportive process that allows managers to leave the organization with the least possible damage to their dignity and self-confidence.

As implied at the outset, a hesitancy to confront management incompetence is universal. Yet the serious ramifications of inaction in a healthcare organization, where the quality of patient care is potentially at risk, cannot be denied. Consequently, executives have a moral obligation to act decisively and, by their own behavior, demonstrate that just as exemplary performance will be properly rewarded, consistently poor performance is unacceptable.

November/December 2005

Must I Maintain Another Person's Promise?

William A. Nelson, PhD

I recently became the CEO of a rural healthcare facility that is experiencing significant financial challenges. During a lengthy tenure, my predecessor implemented several "promises" to employees including a significant bonus for loyal service and formal pension benefits. Tenured employees have come to expect this bonus. Am I ethically obligated to maintain these "promises"?

You raise a question that has legal as well as ethical concerns. Legal counsel should be sought to explore the legal status of prior "promises." I do not believe that nonwritten promises are legally binding even though the promised benefit may have become a general expectation or tradition.

Even in situations where an action or decision is legal, it may still be ethically inappropriate. Therefore, whether or not the promise is legally binding, a decision to accept or not accept your predecessor's promises raises ethical challenges that require a thoughtful, systematic process. Once a decision is made there should be open disclosure of your decision and action, including the reasoning that forms the basis for the decision.

Assuming the promises have become part of the expected retirement benefits, your organizational decision-making process must explore and answer the question: Is there an ethical justification to withdraw a promise that has become imbedded into the facility's retirement tradition?

Because healthcare organizations and individual staff are moral agents, you should start with the premise that basic moral principles or rules ought to be respected unless there is a great deal of weight indicating that you are justified in disregarding the moral principle—in this case, the moral principle is "keep your promise."

The reflection on whether it is justifiable to withdraw the promise hinges on whether the answer to the question produces more harm than good once you have weighed the impact to stakeholders. To answer the question, you will need to explore the cost savings or advantage to the organization if the promised benefit was rescinded. You will also need to carefully assess the cost or harm to the stakeholders such as the employees (both former and current) and the community. How would employee recruitment, retention, and morale be affected? What will be the impact (positive or negative) to the organization's reputation within the community? Are there alternatives to rescinding the promises? To assess both the benefit and harm of all options requires thoughtful analysis and discussion among all relevant stakeholders, such as the chief financial officer, head of human resources, union representative, legal counsel, and of course, employees. You must also consider what approval or communication will be needed with the board.

Living in a small or rural community adds an important contextual dimension to the assessment process because of the overlapping relations between you, the other hospital staff, and retirees. In this situation, it is likely that you, your staff, hospital retirees, and patients are your neighbors and friends—people that you encounter regularly. All of these professional and personal contacts could be affected by the decision.

If the goal is to reduce expenditures, you will need to review other options regarding the overall problem of a financial shortfall. Do the alternatives being considered foster greater or lesser harm? Once alternatives have been identified, including their benefit and harm, you must consider how to rank the options.

Healthcare Executive (2005, Vol. 20, No. 4) stated one such ranking of priorities for healthcare facilities is fostering excellence in patient care, retaining competent and high quality employees necessary for patient care, and maintaining a viable organization. While each of these priorities is essential to deliver quality healthcare, ranking the options requires you to face difficult tradeoffs. Coming to a final decision should include a review of the facility's mission statement.

You might also wish to utilize ACHE's *Code of Ethics* for guidance in your discussions with executives.

Regarding your specific situation, I am reluctant to conclude that breaching your predecessor's promise is appropriate because of the significance of the decision on those impacted. On its surface it would seem that many other, less harmful alternatives, such as a reduction in this bonus, could be identified. However, if there are no other less harmful cost-saving alternatives and the financial survival of your healthcare facility (which is different from improving the facility's business success) is dependent on rescinding the promised benefit, then ending the benefit may morally justify breaking this promise. In the end, facility survival is ethically important because it provides essential healthcare for the community, particularly in areas where access is difficult.

Once a decision is made there should be open discussion about the decision, including the reasoning that formed the basis for the decision. In this example, a communication plan should be developed, including when and how those impacted by the decision will be informed, an explanation of the rationale for the decision, and an opportunity for feedback regarding the decision.

January/February 2006

Evaluating Ethical Fitness

Paul B. Hofmann, DrPH, FACHE

Like every healthcare organization, we expect our senior executives to be role models for ethical behavior. Typically, we assume final candidates would not have achieved their previous success without demonstrating sound moral character, but how can we accurately assess a person's ethical fitness and compatibility with our organization's values?

It is indeed reasonable to expect that well-qualified healthcare professionals would not have been successful if they lacked personal integrity. We would also anticipate that their competence, loyalty, sincerity, honesty, dedication, and ability to meet or exceed performance objectives would be beyond debate. Nonetheless, before making the decision to fill a key management position, there are pitfalls to avoid and a variety of steps to take that will increase the likelihood of a positive outcome for both the candidate and the organization.

PITFALLS TO AVOID

During our careers, we have been interviewed for usually increasingly important positions. Consequently, we have prepared carefully for interviews, trying to predict questions and perhaps rehearsing our responses. In addition, we have developed a list of questions to illustrate our genuine interest in the organization, conveying our curiosity about both its past and its future.

We, like other candidates, want to give answers and ask questions that will please and impress the interviewer. We are confident in our ability, want the job, and may tell ourselves any ambivalence can be resolved when negotiating the final details of the offer. Our ultimate goal is to leave the interviewer with the conviction that no other applicant is as capable as we are. Moreover, if we are less than zealous in employing this strategy, another candidate may be hired. Therefore, while not viewing applicants as inherently disingenuous, interviewers should be reasonably prudent about accepting all responses and inquiries at face value.

A candidate's resume should be scrutinized carefully. If there are employment gaps, the reasons need to be explored. Unfortunately, degrees and credentials still should be confirmed. We continue to read about people with national profiles being fired or forced to resign when "inaccuracies" in their resume have been revealed.

Another pitfall is the potential fallacy of the great reference. When a candidate is asked for references, the person can be expected to provide the names of only those people who will provide positive comments. Even the traditional query about weaknesses or shortcomings may be unlikely to produce much candor. An experienced reference checker will ask both conventional and unconventional questions of the candidate's references. They also should ask for the name of one or two other people who know this person well. Furthermore, they should seek to speak with someone who has a close working relationship with the candidate and is familiar with this individual's moral character but who was not listed as a reference.

STEPS TO ACHIEVE ETHICAL COMPATIBILITY

There are a number of ways to increase the probability that the final candidate and the organization will be ethically compatible.

1. Ask unpredictable questions that probe the candidate's values. For example, "How many people have you fired in the past five years and, if given the opportunity to make the same decisions over again, would you do it any differently?" Another might be, "Describe two or three ethical dilemmas that you encountered in your current or last position and how you dealt with them."

2. Use one of many standardized tests to measure the individual's psychological profile and evaluate this person's responses compared with those of other management team members.

3. Expand the number of individual and group interviews to permit other key members of the organization to explore the candidate's compatibility with the organization.

4. Retain a consultant to assess the candidate's values and their compatibility with those of the organization.

5. Ask the candidate to review three or four brief ethical case studies (one or two paragraphs) and discuss how they should be resolved. These should be tough dilemmas with no obvious "right" answers, requiring the candidate to demonstrate ethical fitness and a rationale for reaching a particular decision. When possible, use scenarios that reflect ethical dilemmas actually faced by your organization in the past.

6. Remember the interviewing process must never be unilateral; it is absolutely essential that the candidate fully understands and supports the organization's values, permitting the candidate to make a well-informed response if a job offer is extended.

Regardless of how comprehensive the evaluation process is, there is no guarantee that the job offer will be made to the ideal candidate. If there are valid misgivings, recruiting more candidates is preferable to selecting someone who is not a good ethical fit. In such cases, the individual and the organization suffer. Ultimately, the leadership team establishes the institution's culture and values. There should be no higher priority than supporting and promoting a management selection process that ensures its culture and values will be enhanced rather than compromised by its newest member.

May/June 2006

Assessing Your Probability for Organizational Success

Paul B. Hofmann, DrPH, FACHE, and Jack R. Schlosser, FACHE

The traditional interviewing process tends to highlight the positive features of both the candidate and the organization. Unfortunately, initial impressions are not always accurate. How can I be sure my personal values and beliefs will be compatible with those of the organization and increase the likelihood that accepting an offer will result in long-term success?

Although there are no guarantees for long-term success, an astute management candidate will realize that vast differences exist among organizations regarding their culture, values, and priorities. For example, some institutions emphasize their focus on improving community health status; teaching hospitals may highlight their academic role; and investor-owned hospitals may underscore their commitment to providing excellent patient care and returning value to their shareholders. The key is finding the right organization to match your own beliefs.

Conventional wisdom dictates that management candidates conduct a thorough evaluation of the organization and its leadership in advance of the first interview. And, of course, even when an executive search firm serves as an intermediary, you have a distinct personal investment to ensure that accepting the position will result in an enduring, productive, and rewarding relationship.

No one disputes the importance of having a comprehensive understanding of your prospective employer. Indeed, evidence reveals that a lack of effective due diligence results in disenchantment and either mutual or unilateral decisions to dissolve the working relationship. Too much reliance is placed on well-polished, eloquent vision, mission, and value statements; strategic plans; and other critical documents. While these materials are certainly relevant and essential background when combined with the typical interviewing process, this review and preliminary positive impressions are still insufficient to make a fully informed decision.

KEY STEPS

To minimize later disappointment and regret, a number of steps can help to maximize a secure and "ethical organizational fit."

- In addition to speaking with those currently employed with the organization, identify former senior executives who have left the organization. Prepare a list of questions that probe attitudes and behaviors to obtain their candid and confidential remarks about its reputation, board, medical staff, management leadership, corporate culture, and values.
- Ask similar questions of others who may have familiarity with the institution, capitalizing on your professional network of colleagues.
- Try to get a sense for turnover statistics within top management ranks, and obtain management's impression of the reasons why people leave.
- Inquire about how success is measured in the organization and its attitude toward risk and failure, perhaps by giving a case description of a situation in which competing values must be reconciled.
- Review the general and business press for articles that may have been published about the organization. Trade magazines,

The Wall Street Journal, BusinessWeek, and similar publications should be researched.

- Think of creative ways to determine if the organization's real behavior, as reflected by its actions and decisions, matches the rhetoric of its well-refined documents.
- Avoid being rushed into a decision. Accept a position only after you have adequate information and are comfortable that you know the organization.
- Consider the chemistry as well as the internal and external dynamics that could impact your role. Assess the likelihood of change in reporting relationships and the management structure.

ADDITIONAL OBSERVATIONS

Consolidations, mergers and affiliations have created many large multisite entities. Consequently, an organization may actually have a number of cultures, although there should be a common set of values shared throughout the organization. The corporate staff may have one orientation and individual hospitals or business units may have another. If a merger has occurred in the recent past, be sensitive to which culture is the dominant one. Focus your efforts on both the overall culture and the unique aspects of the setting in which you will be most involved.

Remember that in the course of a career there are only a limited number of moves that you will likely want to make. Treat each evaluation process with the seriousness that it deserves, and view every potential move as if it is a multiyear commitment.

The allure of a new position with more responsibility and a higher salary in an attractive community can be strong. To ensure that all the professional and personal values are compatible and properly aligned, a wide spectrum of both objective and subjective factors must be examined. A systematic and careful analysis by a candidate should be no less than the intensive scrutiny performed of a candidate by the organization. If both are meticulous and conscientious

in their respective evaluations, the probability of a mutually rewarding long-term relationship will be greatly enhanced.

May/June 2007

The Executive's Role in Malpractice Cases

Paul B. Hofmann, DrPH, FACHE

Progress has been made on improving patient safety and reducing clinical mistakes, but errors happen and, in spite of everything, patients are still harmed. When an error has occurred and a malpractice case is filed, what should be done to maintain the organization's integrity and ensure patients and their families are treated fairly? What values should influence the process?

One of my previous columns ("Responding to Clinical Mistakes," *Healthcare Executive*, September/October 2006) described the need for a comprehensive policy that is consistently applied when a mistake happens. The column also discussed the importance of making a timely disclosure, expressing a sincere apology, explaining steps taken to prevent similar errors, and, when appropriate, indicating an interest in providing proper compensation.

Although studies have reported that the incidence of litigation has been reduced when this approach is taken, individual and institutional healthcare providers will certainly continue to be defendants in malpractice cases. Regrettably, by its very nature, litigation creates an adversarial relationship between the parties. In an eloquent presentation at the National Patient Safety Foundation's 2007 Patient Safety Congress, Susan Sheridan shared her personal experiences following an error that caused permanent brain damage to her newborn son and later the death of her husband due to a failure to communicate malignant spinal cancer pathology.

Mrs. Sheridan's riveting remarks resonated with me for two reasons. First, as a former hospital CEO, I remember a few occasions when our legal counsel asked for my approval to settle a malpractice case in which the hospital had been named, along with physicians, as a codefendant.

After an extensive analysis, sometimes we determined hospital employees were not responsible for the bad outcome, but counsel recommended settlement to avoid adverse publicity and the remote possibility of a higher payment if the case went to trial. In evaluating our legal counsel's recommendation, I thought principally about my administrative and ethical obligations to the organization without devoting much time to my ethical responsibilities to the patient and/or the patient's family.

Second, for a number of years, I have served as an expert witness for both defense and plaintiff attorneys. Consequently, I have reviewed scores of depositions, given my own deposition and testified in court. This experience has given me a deeper appreciation for the nature and politics of malpractice cases. Even more important, it has provided greater insight into why patients and their families pursue litigation and what happens to them when they do.

Mrs. Sheridan's presentation was included in the July/August 2007 issue of *Patient Safety and Quality Healthcare.* The article, "We're Not Your Enemy," was coauthored with Martin Hatlie, JD, president of Partnership for Patient Safety. It should be required reading for every healthcare executive. In the article, the authors noted that medical-legal research has found that the existing tort system undercompensates the majority of patients and families who have suffered medical error. Assuming the validity of this finding, what are some of the noneconomic costs that cannot be quantified?

Despite impressions to the contrary, it is anger, not greed, that drives most malpractice lawsuits. Among other factors, this anger is usually driven by denials that a mistake occurred; the lack of timely disclosure and apology; a refusal to meet with a patient, family members, or both to discuss an error; the unwillingness of the hospital, physicians, and perhaps others responsible for the mistake to cooperate in providing a fair settlement; and a general sense that the organization was insensitive to the patient or family's needs.

So what can happen as the result of subsequent litigation? In Mrs. Sheridan's case, it seemed like a never-ending nightmare. She said:

> We learned with great alarm and extreme disappointment that litigation is a "win-at-all-costs blame game" that it is wildly inconsistent and deviously strategic and which rarely makes our healthcare system safer. We learned that expert testimony could be bought, that medical records could disappear, and that patients and family members were often pressured to keep quiet in the settlement process. We witnessed a culture of collusion and cover up.

LESSONS FOR HEALTHCARE ORGANIZATIONS

Let us suppose a hospital does everything possible to prevent clinical errors and works conscientiously with patients and family members to reach an amicable settlement when a mistake has been made. Despite these efforts, a malpractice suit has been filed. How should the organization respond?

Typically, the institution's insurance carrier retains a law firm to defend the case and, unless it is accompanied by extensive publicity, the hospital CEO's personal involvement may be quite minimal. Mrs. Sheridan's poignant story suggests her situation was not unique, and my own experience confirms that senior management frequently has little or no participation in any aspect of the defense process.

Risk managers, insurance carriers, and outside counsel are motivated to win each case and minimize every settlement. Strategically, these are their objectives, and implicitly they are management's expectations as well. The legal and financial value of this strategy is obvious, but is it consistent with an organization's ethical values?

Most hospital value statements are created to capture and convey the institution's ethical principles and commitments and usually highlight the importance of excellence, respect, integrity, dignity, compassion, stewardship, justice, and similar virtues. If healthcare organizations are genuinely dedicated to fulfilling these virtues they must be consistently reflected in the way malpractice cases are handled. For many hospitals, this will require re-examining who is overseeing cases and what ethical template is used to assess how they are being managed.

The direct involvement of the CEO in all malpractice cases may have a valuable benefit. Engaging the CEO could possibly temper some of the inevitable adversarial dimensions of litigation and contribute to more timely and reasonable settlements.

At least annually, hospital CEOs should be giving a report to the board on malpractice cases and their outcomes. In making and discussing this report, they should consider Mrs. Sheridan's closing remarks: "Remember that people who experience medical errors are not just dollar figures. We are your loved ones. We are you."

May/June 2008

The Use and Misuse of Incentives

Paul B. Hofmann, DrPH, FACHE

We know financial and nonfinancial incentives are designed to encourage specific personal behaviors and to achieve both individual and organizational performance goals. What steps can be taken to avoid or minimize their unintended consequences?

Beginning in early childhood, everyone learns the power of incentives, disincentives and sanctions. Their unquestionable influence shaped our daily behavior, attitudes and decisions. As children our actions were often the result of the rewards, praise, applause, criticism, disapproval, and perhaps even ridicule we received.

We carry these lessons into adulthood and into our professional careers where we become increasingly aware of how and why the proper alignment of incentives at each level of the organization is essential to producing positive outcomes. The type of organization, its tax status, position in the market, form of governance, leadership, and culture all set the stage for either implicit or explicit incentives for both individual and group behavior. Unfortunately, and often too late, many organizations also discover the "dark side" of incentives.

INCENTIVES' DARK SIDE

Without proper alignment and oversight, incentives can inadvertently promote unethical behavior. When results are more valued than honesty and pressure intensifies to generate better outcomes, it is not surprising to witness an increase in unethical behavior. This behavior can be demonstrated in the distortion, manipulation, or concealment of data to improve

- financial results;
- pay-for-performance rewards;
- internal and external comparative analyses relative to finance or patient care;
- public perceptions of the organization;
- job performance of either individuals or work groups;
- support by employees and medical staff for organizational change or CEO decisions;
- budget controls that affect jobs, services and/or physician income; or
- arrangements with private health plans or government payment programs.

Historically, hospital payment programs are a prime example of the power of incentives to discourage efficiency under cost-based reimbursement (1965 to 1983) and then to encourage cutting even necessary costs under DRG-based reimbursement. Similarly, physician payment policies have been criticized for encouraging unwarranted visits and procedures under fee-for-service payment and discouraging legitimate services under managed care, particularly capitation.

But incentives of all kinds remain a popular instrument of management, so it is worth considering what happens when they are used unwisely. For example, unrealistic budget targets, in addition to stimulating possible financial fraud and abuse, may be set too high in order to meet an income goal or too low for the actual volume of work to be done, damaging staff morale and quality of care. Block scheduling of outpatient visits can improve efficiency while lengthening patient waiting times.

If there is an incentive to reduce incident reports, patient and employee safety will be compromised if adverse events are then underreported. When employees see incentives that are counterproductive, unevenly applied, or inadequate, they become cynical about subsequent initiatives.

Sandeep Jauhar, MD, notes in a September 9, 2008, *New York Times* article that too little attention has been devoted to the pitfalls of judging physician performance by surgical report cards and compliance with clinical guidelines. According to one study, the proliferation of surgical report cards has encouraged cardiac surgeons to accept only relatively healthy patients.

Jauhar also references the Medicare requirement that antibiotics be administered to a pneumonia patient within six hours of arriving at the hospital. He indicates physicians cannot always diagnose pneumonia that quickly, so now the overuse of antibiotics in emergency rooms has led to a rise in antibiotic-resistant bacteria and antibiotic-associated infections.

RECOMMENDATIONS

To minimize the unintended consequences of incentives:

1. Build a foundation for ethical behavior. Select the right people for the board, recruit morally conscientious employees, and appoint highly principled medical staff members. Make discussion of ethics a more prominent topic in board, management, and medical staff meetings.
2. Consider the ways an incentive could be abused. Recognize that an employee's need for job security and/or advancement can trump appropriate conduct, especially when this person feels vulnerable or is overly ambitious.

3. Think imaginatively about the full range of potential unintended consequences of a specific program or policy. Challenge a diverse group of staff members to state what negative developments could possibly result from implementing a particular incentive designed to stimulate only positive outcomes. For instance, is it possible that improvements in infection control or surgical outcomes could be publicized prematurely without verification, or that adverse reports could be concealed, delayed, or downplayed?

3. Make a commitment to complete transparency by sharing information fully, quickly, and factually—an incentive to promote accountability is hypocritical and unethical if the commitment is fulfilled only when there is good news to share. Help board members avoid overreaction when bad news is expressed openly, even if they fear it will harm the reputation of the organization or worry the medical staff.

4. Incorporate elements designed to minimize and discourage inappropriate behavior within incentive plans.

5. Analyze an incentive's positive and negative effects on patients, which may raise or lower perceptions of the organization's integrity and ethics. If families have to endure bankruptcy or forgo needed medical treatment because of a provider's unreasonable pricing policies or collection methods formed by the use of incentives, the community will not be comforted by the organization's claim that "all healthcare institutions do this."

The proper use of incentives can have a positive impact on quality of care and the bottom line. By fully considering all the undesirable consequences of incentives, executives can avoid higher costs and potential embarrassment for the organization. More importantly, patients and the public will be the ultimate beneficiaries.

January/February 2009

PART II:

ORGANIZATIONAL

ETHICS ISSUES

ORGANIZATIONAL ETHICS REFERS to ethical management and business activities requiring deliberations, decisions, and actions by leaders of the organization. Organizational ethics includes the positions and practices that define an organization internally and externally. This section focuses on an array of ethical challenges within the context of the healthcare organization that need reflection and resolution. An organization's vision, mission, value statements, and code of ethics help to create the organization's culture. However, policies, procedures, and guidelines need to be developed, implemented, monitored, and clarified to foster an ethical organization. This section addresses many specific issues regarding organizational decisions that establish ethical standards of practice.

Ensuring Fair
Termination Procedures

Paul B. Hofmann, DrPH, FACHE

WHEN HEALTHCARE EXECUTIVES are faced with a termination decision, a number of issues arise. Although many of these issues are legal ones, a number of critical ethical considerations must be made as well.

The potential for violating ethical standards exists both before and following an employee's termination. Throughout the discharge process, it is the healthcare executive's responsibility to act in the organization's best interest while ensuring that the employee is treated fairly.

Because the imposition of any sanction, particularly termination, is uncomfortable for all parties, there is an undeniable tendency to procrastinate and rationalize reasons for doing so. However, neither the organization nor the individual involved is well served by a failure to confront a discharge situation in a timely manner.

The organization's effectiveness is compromised by the performance of a marginal employee. The credibility of the manager is damaged by a perceived weakness to act promptly. And, the employees working with or being supervised by the individual in question are certainly affected adversely. Further, if the decision to act is made late and a wrongful termination charge is filed, ethically and legally the decision maker is vulnerable if performance discussions and related events have not been documented.

In addition to facing discharge decisions regarding poor-performing individuals, healthcare executives continue to gain painful experience in making layoff decisions. Because personnel cutbacks may become increasingly necessary, a comprehensive plan for conducting layoffs is essential.

The ethical issues involved in laying off healthcare staff are no different than those for employees in other fields. Therefore, the plan should emphasize such fundamentals as

- the provision of timely, accurate information (control rumors by keeping personnel informed),
- fulfillment of salary and benefit commitments, and
- meaningful outplacement assistance.

It is critical to remember that whether terminating an employee or planning, announcing, and implementing layoffs, the healthcare executive's actions will have profound and pervasive implications not only for these individuals, but for the staff who remain. The need for ethical sensitivity in these matters cannot be overstated.

TERMINATION FOLLOW-UP

Virtually all senior executives have, at one time or another, experienced ambivalence about the type and extent of reference information to release about terminated employees. Confirming only the dates of employment may minimize time, energy, and possible liability, but, under most circumstances, taking such a stance is unreasonable and unnecessary. Honesty and relevancy are the underlying principles that should guide the release of all information. If these two criteria are met, an executive will have complied with a professional and ethical obligation to be responsive.

Obviously, when a discharge has been contentious, particular caution should be exercised in answering questions. As a general guideline, if the truth might harm the candidate's job prospects, the information can be provided if it was shared previously with the discharged employee and, preferably, documented.

Restrictions on a reference are greatest when a formal, written agreement with the discharged employee specifies what can be released. In such a situation, no discretion or judgments are entailed; the legal requirements are clear, and no ethical dilemma exists.

January/February 1994

Serving and Competing Ethically

Paul B. Hofmann, DrPH, FACHE

Regardless of whether a provider is not-for-profit or investor-owned, it has a formal mission statement and may have formal vision and value statements. However, if these documents fail to actually guide organizational and individual decision making, they are more than empty and meaningless rhetoric—they are symptoms of professional hypocrisy.

At a time when there is growing awareness that community and population-based health planning hold the best promise for improving community health status, many organizations are revisiting their mission statements.

At the same time, the growing influence of managed care, particularly capitation, has fostered sometimes fierce competition among providers. Even in those geographic areas where managed care has a relatively small penetration, excess bed capacity related to shorter lengths of stay and more outpatient surgery has stimulated aggressive marketing and advertising programs.

Serving and competing ethically in this environment is not impossible, but the challenge should not be underestimated. Promoting the best interest of the organization and serving the public's best interest are not always compatible objectives. For example, although unlikely in most situations, it is conceivable that a community's need might be best served if a hospital were to close. Similarly, an exceptionally successful marketing campaign that generates a significant increase in admission to one hospital could do so at the cost of irreparably compromising a competing hospital's ability to meet the needs of a largely medically indigent population.

Effective, ethical leaders are those who can sustain a delicate balance; they are able to achieve financial targets while maximizing community benefit. To help your healthcare organization meet its commitment to serve and compete ethically:

- Take measures to ensure that your mission, vision, and values statements are understood by every staff member and that decisions and actions are consistent with these statements.
- Ask yourself what the potential negative effects on the community will be and how they can be mitigated before embarking on competitive strategies.
- Avoid the temptation to excuse inefficient business practices by rationalizing that a not-for-profit organization need not adopt progressive and perhaps even aggressive policies and procedures.
- Actively engage board, management, and physician participation in any significant changes affecting the organization's image or role in the community.
- Evaluate the possible noneconomic as well as economic ramifications of reducing or eliminating programs or services.

Competition in healthcare is not inherently bad. Ultimately, we must remember that competition, like any other concept, can be distorted or abused. The fundamental ethical imperative for healthcare executives, regardless of institutional ownership, is to optimize the benefits of competition for the community as well as the organization.

July/August 1995

Beyond the Margin

Michael G. Daigneault, Esq.

As the CEO of a not-for-profit healthcare system, I am struggling to find a balance between my responsibility to my organization and to my community. Obviously, my system is expected to operate in the black; it also, however, is committed to providing care to the poor and underserved. How do I balance these two—seemingly contradictory—responsibilities?

Often, in the examples used to teach ethical decision making, the inherent conflicts in the ethical dilemmas are relatively simple. For example, value conflicts are often demonstrated with hypothetical questions such as: Is it acceptable to steal a loaf of bread to feed a starving child? Is it okay to tell someone that she "looks wonderful" when her age or illness is making her look less than terrific? In these cases, the dilemma is quite clear.

In the case stated here, there appears to be a dilemma: fiscal responsibility versus community service. However, the underlying question is whether these "seemingly contradictory responsibilities" are, in fact, in conflict.

The issue is that healthcare systems must foster their overall financial well-being while maintaining certain services to the community that do not in themselves produce a positive revenue stream. Segments of healthcare such as emergency services, neonatal care, mental health services, and yes, care for the poor, are not particularly cost-effective. That there is sometimes little or no margin for these particular services, however, does not mean they should be eliminated.

At the same time, operating "in the black" is an essential obligation of any healthcare organization. As the Sisters of Mercy are frequently noted as saying, "no margin, no mercy." This does not mean that margin is—or should be—the raison d'être of a healthcare organization. It does suggest, however, that "margin" is a necessary, but insufficient, precondition to success. It is the raw material of caring for the poor and underserved.

As with any of the community's other competing needs, the economic burden that any healthcare system must bear to help the underserved must be fairly and appropriately balanced and managed. But it is a burden that should and must be borne.

Why? Because the bond of trust that exists between healthcare providers and the communities they serve goes far beyond mandated legal or business obligations—individuals have no other viable choice but to depend on the existing healthcare system in their community. Because of that special trust, healthcare providers must conduct all their medical and business activities in a caring and ethical manner.

This argues for the proposition that all healthcare organizations bear a collective responsibility to meet the healthcare needs of the communities they serve. There will likely always be a dynamic tension between the needs of a community and the capacity of any healthcare organization, hospital, or healthcare system to meet those needs. But this does not preclude a healthcare organization from meeting its own business and financial objectives.

In other words, there may not be an ethical dilemma here, at least not at the macro level. At the highest level, these values—financial responsibility and community service—are not in conflict; rather, one is a precondition needed to support the other.

There is often tension between these values, however, as there never seems to be enough money to do all that we could or would do to serve society. Every organization has at one time maintained that it could do more if only it had more time, people, and money.

At the macro level, we know that not everyone can get everything they want every time they want it. But, that is little solace as we agonize over whether to commit resources to meet a given individual's needs. The best we can strive to accomplish, as we balance both margin and mercy, is to allocate our limited resources in ways that optimize the value we give to society—that do the most good for the greatest number.

In practical terms, doing so may, in some cases, limit our services to the necessities of saving lives and easing pain. We may desire to do more, to add quality to the lives of those we serve, not just longevity. We may wish to save the leg, not just the life. We may wish to heal the wound and leave no scar. But we do not get all that we wish for. We cannot save the leg if doing so costs another's life. It is the fundamental lesson of triage: finite resources spread over a great need.

We may despair and wish it were not so, but it is. How do we balance what at first glance appear to be contradictory responsibilities? As best we can—with humanity and humility. But, balance them we must. If we fail to provide for either margin or mercy today, we will fail to provide for both of them tomorrow.

November/December 1997

Reconciling Conflicts of Interest

Gordon C. Hunt, MD, MBA

The part-time medical director in my organization is responsible for overseeing a medical quality assurance program. However, he is also a specialist who relies on referrals from colleagues and is worried about alienating them by reporting their variances from approved clinical protocols. How should both he and our organization address this conflict of interest?

There are a number of questions that should be addressed in this situation:

1. Is the quality assurance program appropriately addressing variances as an opportunity to improve care, or does the process contribute to a "culture of blame"?
2. Does the medical director have guidelines from the medical staff and the facility that clearly delineate when variances should be reported to the medical staff peer review process?
3. Does the medical director have the opportunity to use outside consultants and independent third parties to guide decision making?
4. When necessary, is the medical director willing and able to fulfill the primary responsibility of the job: to protect patient

safety, even at the risk of upsetting colleagues who refer patients?

CREATING A CULTURE OF IMPROVEMENT VS. A CULTURE OF BLAME

We should first clarify the difference between a quality assurance program and the punitive aspects of the medical staff peer review process. Modern quality assurance programs identify areas that can be improved in the delivery of care, rather than assigning blame for less-than-optimal outcomes. Peer review is a formal process in which a physician's performance is assessed by the medical staff; in the past, this process has focused on poor performance. The historical use of the peer review process to discipline physicians for poor performance has contributed to a "culture of blame" in many organizations.

In the context of your situation, the difference between these two approaches is important because reporting variances from a clinical protocol need not be disciplinary—in fact, it shouldn't be. There are often good reasons to deviate from a clinical protocol, and even when the protocol should have been followed, an evaluation of the situation and the process can offer real opportunities to learn and improve performance. By distinguishing quality assurance from the punitive aspects of the peer review process, you can facilitate the improvement process and remove much of the conflict that concerns your medical director.

Most errors in medicine are due to the failure of a process, rather than the failure of an individual. Focusing your quality review program on process improvement and identifying and preventing errors will eliminate many of the conflicts your medical director fears—and it will help you develop a culture of process improvement. Then, the medical director can do his or her job with less potential conflict with colleagues. At the core of the issue is whether the quality review process has moved past the "culture of blame" into the modern era of performance improvement.

FULFILLING RESPONSIBILITIES

This doesn't mean that your medical director won't identify serious situations in which a physician's performance is substandard and requires intervention. On occasion, at least, the medical director risks raising the ire of colleagues upon whom he or she depends for referrals. The key question you must ask when you discover that a physician's performance endangers patients' safety or compromises their care is simply, "Whom are we ultimately trying to protect?" If a physician's performance impairs the delivery of care and puts a patient at risk, the medical director's obligation is clear: The first and primary duty is to protect patients.

If your medical director is so personally conflicted about his or her ability to work effectively in this process, either the position itself is not outlined properly or the wrong person has been selected for the job. If the medical director's role hasn't been properly defined, you should outline the specific responsibilities of the medical director and how that person relates organizationally to the medical staff peer review process. The organization should clearly delineate which issues merit the attention of the peer review process and which are part of the ongoing quality assurance program of the hospital and medical staff.

For example, the quality review process may track returns to the operating room. For surgical procedures that rarely require a return to the operating room, the medical staff can dictate that when a return to the operating room does occur, it is automatically referred to the peer review process. This policy takes the judgment and subjectivity out of the hands of the medical director heading the quality assurance program by mandating that the medical director report the case to the peer review process. In this way, the decision is already made before the specific situation occurs, greatly simplifying the role of the medical director.

If your medical staff is small and few physicians are qualified to oversee the quality assurance program in your organization, consider using external consultants to supplement and support the medical director. This is often an effective means for dealing with conflict because it shares a difficult decision with an external party who has the skills and experience needed, but who is not in direct competition with or dependent on referrals from other physicians in the organization.

If the medical director's role has been appropriately defined but the medical director is unable to confront colleagues when appropriate, then the situation needs to be resolved by filling that position with someone who can work successfully through the conflict.

November/December 2002

A Community
Approach to Free Care

William D. Petasnick , FACHE

While our community hospital is committed to providing free care to those in need, in trying to fulfill this part of our mission we are reaching our limits financially. How should we address our free care obligation in a financial context while maintaining an ethical position?

In my experience, to best address this issue we should begin with the premise that providing healthcare to the uninsured and under-insured is a shared community responsibility. And the provision of care to such individuals is a social benefit, whose costs should be shouldered broadly. Therefore, the question you raise poses ethical issues for our entire society, not just your hospital. All participants in the healthcare system—including providers, insurers, employers, and governments at all levels (national, state, county, and local)—have a role to play in providing indigent care. Your ethical responsibility as a hospital is to serve as a catalyst to engage all other participants and encourage the need for "fair share" participation by all.

As president of Froedtert Memorial Lutheran Hospital in Milwaukee, I learned firsthand that a public-private approach to indigent care can help maintain the public safety net. In 1980, Froedtert Hospital was created as a result of a compromise under Wisconsin's Certificate of Need laws. Under that agreement, Froedtert entered a unique relationship with Milwaukee County's Doyne Hospital in which the organizations worked together as "two half hospitals." The county hospital retained the trauma center, oncology, obstetrics, and other services; furthermore, this hospital fulfilled the county's responsibility to provide indigent care. Froedtert—a private hospital— became the center for neurosciences, solid organ transplantation, and medical/surgical subspecialties. The hospitals agreed to cooperate with the joint goal of "improvement and enhancement of medical care in the community."

The arrangement, albeit complicated and cumbersome, continued until the mid-1990s, when Doyne simply could not survive the pressure of being the sole provider of free care in the area. At that time, county officials began discussions with Froedtert that led to the closure of Doyne Hospital and merged the assets of the county hospital with Froedtert's to form one organization. It is important to note that Milwaukee County did not abdicate its role in providing healthcare to the uninsured. Rather, the county opted to become a purchaser of services utilizing a capped financial model that was a combination of county levy dollars and state block grant funds, including federal disproportionate share funding. However, as Milwaukee County had experienced, the need for care exceeded the available funding, and we knew that Froedtert could not stay viable if we simply tried to pick up where Doyne left off as the next indigent care provider. Thus, Froedtert took the lead in forging a community approach to providing care to the uninsured.

In 1996, Froedtert—in conjunction with three other federally qualified health centers in the area and the Medical College of Wisconsin—proposed a program aimed at establishing an integrated delivery system that would achieve greater coordination between community-based clinics and acute care centers for indigent residents. Some of the group's objectives included

- integrating multiple health and wellness services at readily accessible community locations;

- reallocating resources from acute care to health promotion, prevention, and early intervention;
- developing extended-hours, urgent care sites as an alternative to the inappropriate use of hospital emergency departments;
- establishing a management system capable of monitoring resource utilization and making timely operational adjustments;
- broadening the responsibility for indigent care to include both public and private institutions and resources; and
- demonstrating cost-effective care and prudent use of public dollars to encourage ongoing county support.

Phase one of the program was intended to transfer the preventive/primary healthcare services from Froedtert to the three other health centers over a 12-month period while establishing the systems needed to meet the above objectives. The second phase would expand the program to additional providers, including more clinics, hospitals, and specialty providers, to achieve a wider disbursement of care and easier access to care for patients.

The proposal was approved in March 1997. Since then, the program has grown to include 15 clinics with a total of 27 sites, each with its own network of providers for specialty care, ancillary pharmacy, home health, and inpatient care—with all 10 hospitals in the county participating. Milwaukee County contracts directly with each community clinic for the full array of services with the exception of inpatient, emergency, and trauma care provided through hospitals. Regarding hospital care, Milwaukee County opted to contract with the three major health systems on behalf of the individual hospitals within each system.

What has happened to the patients previously served by the county hospital? According to the Planning Council, an independent organization hired by Milwaukee County to analyze data, the closure of Doyne Hospital did not result in a disruption of care to the uninsured. In fact, access has improved due to the many sites of care now available. While the number of individuals served since 1996 has remained constant over the years, the percentage of care provided by Froedtert versus the percentage of care provided by community clinics and other hospitals changed substantially. For example, in January of 1996, Froedtert provided 94 percent of indigent care; by 2001, Froedtert accounted for only 28 percent of the county's indigent care budget. These decreases in utilization at Froedtert were accompanied by increases in the usage of community-based clinics and nine other hospitals from virtually no services in 1996 to 40 percent of the 2001 budget. As these data show, the private and public sectors have been able to establish an effective partnership to meet a community need.

The ranks of the uninsured are going to continue to grow. But while hospitals have a responsibility to provide care to community members who are in need, they also have a responsibility to remain viable. To abdicate free care in a way that threatens the viability of one healthcare provider can only be viewed as community harm— no matter what other benefits are provided. If, as a single provider, you recognize that your organization may not be able to do it all, then you have an ethical responsibility to bring other community participants to the table to share the responsibility with you.

January/February 2002

Addressing Bioterrorism

John M. Haas, PhD, STL

High expectations have been placed on our nation's healthcare organizations to respond effectively to the results of terrorist activity, specifically bioterrorist attacks. Are there any ethical issues that may not be obvious? What challenges do they pose?

In the wake of the terrible assaults of September 11, 2001, on New York and Washington, DC, a bioterrorist attack was launched against segments of the U.S. population. The anthrax attack vividly demonstrated the vulnerability of our country to bioterrorism—whether from distant or domestic enemies—and awakened a series of complex ethical issues for healthcare organizations and their leaders to consider.

PREPARING FOR AN ATTACK THROUGH VACCINATIONS

Currently, much debate swirls around the U.S. government's proposal to vaccinate healthcare workers, military personnel, other first-responders, and eventually the general public against smallpox. The Centers for Disease Control and Prevention and the National Institute of Allergic and Infectious Disease have categorized smallpox—as well as anthrax, plague, tularemia, botulism toxin, and hemorrhagic fever—as Category A agents, meaning that they are the "weaponized" biological agents most likely to be used by terrorists. Although smallpox is virtually nonexistent in this country, it is considered one of the most dangerous potential biological weapons because it is easily transmitted from person to person. Highly contagious, the virus kills 30 percent of its victims when unchecked by inoculations.

The severe threat smallpox poses if wielded in an attack prompted President Bush's vaccination proposal. Mandatory orders to inoculate 500,000 military personnel are already under way, and the president was himself vaccinated as commander in chief. While vaccinations for the general public are voluntary—but recommended—the government hopes that the bulk of U.S. civilians will choose to be vaccinated by 2004.

Vaccinations take place with a live virus, which can lead to some severe and occasional life-threatening complications. One to two people out of one million may actually die as a result of complications from the vaccinations—generally individuals with compromised immune systems. Some hospitals and healthcare organizations have refused to have their workers vaccinated because they do not consider the risk of a smallpox bioterrorist attack to be as great as the risk resulting from the vaccination itself. For one, they have weighed the risk that their staff might suffer injury or death—however unlikely—as the result of vaccinations and do not believe that the benefit outweighs the potential risk. Secondly, many of these organizations are concerned about the chances that the disease will spread from an inoculated person to a person who is not immunized—thus endangering the very patients that healthcare professionals are entrusted to serve.

Those supporting smallpox vaccines counter that newly inoculated staff can be excluded from the workplace for two to three weeks to avoid the risk of spreading the disease; however, this is truly a financial impossibility for most hospitals. The complex decision regarding smallpox vaccinations confronts healthcare leaders with a variety of choices, including: Which healthcare workers should be inoculated? Can the hospital afford it? Can the hospital assume the risk of liability if there are adverse reactions to the inoculation?

RESPONDING TO AN ATTACK WITH AVAILABLE RESOURCES

First-Responders

Should a bioterrorist attack occur, public health authorities will be confronted with ethical decisions about who should first receive vaccines against a dangerous biological agent. This determination will likely be made on the basis of whether individuals are in a position to render a public service in safeguarding the health of the community. For example, those receiving prophylaxis or treatment first would probably include healthcare workers and their staff; emergency medical service personnel; firefighters and police officers; coroners and medical examiners; key public officials, such as governors and their public health officers; members of emergency management teams; and perhaps even those who are responsible for water, power, and communications systems. After these individuals have been treated or protected, decisions would need to be made about other segments of the population. Those with greater responsibility for the common good would likely be assured of treatment or protection first, so that they might work for the benefit of greater numbers. In fact, certain lives may actually be deemed to be of greater social value in the sense that the general population depends on the good health of those individuals and their capacity to make decisions for the sake of the greater number of people.

Afflicted Patients

And what about the individuals who have been infected with the smallpox virus in the face of a terrorist attack and seek treatment from our healthcare organizations? In circumstances of biological warfare, decisions may have to be made as to who should receive treatment, especially if large segments of the population are infected and medical resources are overwhelmed. Judgments may have to be made about when to remove a ventilator from a person who is dying to assist another who may have a chance for survival. Antibiotics may be available only to those who would have a reasonable likelihood of responding to the treatment. Situations could easily be envisioned that would require quarantine for certain elements of the population, and the state might even have to dictate how the corpses of loved ones should be disposed.

In the current situation in which the U.S. finds itself, public authorities may need to assume extraordinary powers for the sake of public safety. Laws and directives may be passed that restrict the liberties of citizens more so than would be the case in periods of peace. Such determinations are the responsibility of those who bear civil authority, which is ultimately exercised for the sake of the common good. In Washington and across the country, public health agencies have been drawing up guidelines for action in the event of further biological attacks—guidelines that would admittedly curtail certain exercises of individual autonomy.

Already some bioethicists have expressed concern that the "hard-won" recognition of patient autonomy might be diminished with appeals to the needs of the community to protect itself from the spread of deadly or debilitating diseases. For example, public health officials might have to know the identities of those with whom an infected person has been in contact. In other circumstances, this might be viewed as an invasion of privacy or a violation of confidentiality. But in the face of the mortal danger of the spread of a highly contagious viral infection such as smallpox, the sick person would have a grave moral obligation to reveal the names of those with whom he or she had recently been in contact—even if this led to those individuals being quarantined.

Public officials are clearly charged by their office to protect and promote the common good of society while respecting the rights of individual citizens. As long as the natural rights of citizens are not violated, priority should be given to the common good so that the well-being of the largest number of citizens can be advanced as far as possible. In such circumstances, sentimentality cannot direct public or institutional policy; instead, those policies should be guided by reasonable judgments about the benefits that can be derived for the common good from the decisions of those in authority.

May/June 2003

Health Literacy: An Ethical Responsibility

Gloria G. Mayer, RN, EdD, FAAN, and Michael Villaire, MSLM

Providers in our healthcare network distribute patient information sheets, ask patients if they understand their treatment options, and call back after the visit to ensure the patient is doing well. Lately, we've been hearing a lot of talk about health literacy. How far does my organization's responsibility go in addressing the health literacy of our patients?

The short answer to this question is that your responsibility goes as far as it needs to go to ensure that your patients are equipped to make truly informed, appropriate choices about their care. Passing out information sheets, asking questions, and making follow-up calls are excellent if the patient can read and comprehend the materials you have given them. If patients cannot read, then the head-nodding and affirmative answers that patients respond with are often provided out of shame, rather than understanding. The impact of low health literacy on patients and the healthcare organizations that serve them is far-reaching—as is our ethical responsibility as healthcare executives to ease it.

THE IMPACT OF LOW HEALTH LITERACY

Many definitions exist, but simply put, health literacy is the ability to understand healthcare information—such as instructions regarding prescriptions, informed consent documents, health information sheets, and insurance forms—and to use that information to make decisions about one's healthcare. Given that more than 90 million Americans are either functionally illiterate or unable to read above a fifth-grade level, it is astounding that most patient information material is written at a tenth-grade reading level or higher. Furthermore, much of it is peppered with mystifying medical jargon and terminology that reflects our increasingly complex healthcare system and treatment options.

The implications of low health literacy for our nation's healthcare system are staggering. According to the U.S. Department of Adult Education, poor literacy may lead to the improper use of medication, rehospitalization, birth defects, incurable cancer that may have been detected earlier if the patient had understood its seriousness and implications, and other problems. The cost of low health literacy in human suffering is immeasurable.

On an operational level, low health literacy has a negative impact on healthcare costs. A study conducted by the National Academy on an Aging Society concluded that low health literacy skills increase annual healthcare expenditures by $73 billion (in 1998 healthcare dollars). The study found that the main source of these expenditures was longer hospital stays; ineffective use of prescriptions or misunderstandings about treatment plans also may have financial consequences. Healthcare providers and those who finance them—such as Medicare, Medicaid, and employers—assume part of the financial burden by sharing it with patients who have low health literacy skills.

THE ETHICAL DIMENSIONS OF IMPROVING HEALTH LITERACY

The responsibilities of healthcare executives have multiple ethical dimensions, one of which is to their organization as a business concern. On this front alone, healthcare executives have an obligation to improve the health literacy of their patients. Operationally, it makes good business sense. But is promoting health literacy only a fiduciary responsibility to our organizations and their shareholders?

Certainly not. Healthcare executives have an obligation to attend to the best interests of every person served by our organizations. Our primary duty is to protect patients, to be their advocates, and to be stewards of good health for our communities. Since patients with low literacy levels are more likely to report poor health conditions, as found by the National Center for the Study of Adult Learning and Literacy, then working to improve the health literacy of the underserved and vulnerable members of our communities is an ethical imperative. One could argue that accountability lies with the patient. In the past, healthcare organizations have labeled patients who did not follow the instructions given to them by their providers as "noncompliant." But if patients cannot follow instructions because they cannot understand them, accusing them of non-compliance is unfair.

As a solution, some patient advocates suggest that healthcare organizations route resources into literacy programs to ensure that every child grows into an adult who can read at a tenth-grade level. While partnering with communities in supporting literacy programs is an effective long-term solution, our hospitals and health systems are flooded today with adult patients who cannot understand healthcare information. Although simple literacy tests exist, their application in the healthcare setting is problematic and ultimately unnecessary—if your organization treats all patients by providing easy-to-understand and easy-to-use materials. Any of the following ideas can help you improve the health literacy of your patients:

- Review your own health information—be it provided via the Internet, printed brochures, or conversation—to ensure it communicates easily. Organizations like the Institute for Healthcare Advancement can point you toward sources that can help you evaluate the reading level of your materials. Reduce the discrepancies between the readability levels of patient education materials and reading levels of the audience for which they are intended by rewriting them at a lower level. Be especially attentive to the use of medical jargon by making sure that words used between providers and patients are straightforward and simple. Nearly everyone understands bleeding, high blood pressure, and cancer. Not everyone understands hemorrhage, hypertension, and carcinoma or metastases.

- Use illustrations to increase patient comprehension, especially among low-literate populations. Limited literacy also affects listening and speaking abilities, not just reading ability. Decontextualized medical language can be difficult to understand.
- Provide education that will help your physicians develop patient communication skills. Physicians should be asking patients to explain a diagnosis or treatment in their own words. They should also ask them exactly how they plan on taking their medication. It shouldn't surprise anyone that "take when you awaken" or "take with food" may be misinterpreted.

The healthcare organization's function is to diagnose, explain, and treat. The patient's responsibility is to listen, ask questions, choose treatment options, follow a prescription regimen, and make appropriate lifestyle choices. When it works properly, a partnership between the patient and provider is a powerful alliance. But if communication breaks down in the partnership, then the outcome is poor and the burden upon the patient and the healthcare system is only increased. How far do we need to go to ensure that our patients understand? As far as necessary to ensure that they understand.

July/August 2003

Your Board and Conflicts of Interest

John G. King, FACHE

In most communities, business leaders (bankers, insurance agency owners, lawyers, etc.) commonly serve as board members for local healthcare organizations. Must a board nominee agree to cut all business relationships with a healthcare organization and promise not to bid on future business as a condition of candidacy? What issues should be considered in evaluating board candidates and resolving potential conflicts of interest?

In its recent publication "Fundamental Fiduciary Duties of the Nonprofit Healthcare Director," the Governance Institute identifies oversight and the related duties of care, loyalty, and obedience to corporate purpose (see diagram) as the fundamental fiduciary duties of a healthcare organization's board of directors. To fulfill their duty of loyalty, board members are obligated to disclose situations that "may present a potential for conflict with the corporation's mission, as well as a duty to avoid competition with, and appropriation of the assets of, the corporation." With this in mind, we can examine your last question first.

Hospital and health system boards are usually composed of three types of directors: external directors from the community, physicians from within the organization, and executive officers from within the organization. Conflicts of interest can occur among directors in all

The Duty of Oversight (Diagrammed)

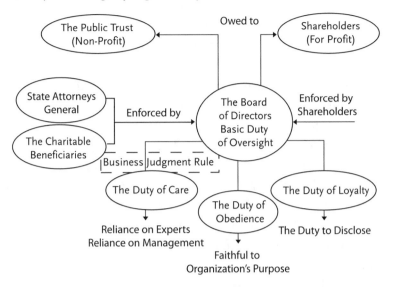

Source: Virginia Mason Medical Center. Used with permission.

three categories, but the approaches for dealing with them are similar. To guard against conflicts of interest, a number of preventative measures can be taken, including the following:

- **Develop a formal policy.** Create a policy statement that describes precisely how your directors are to discharge their duties in the context of loyalty to the healthcare organization. This policy should be clear not only to potential members of the board prior to their appointment, but also to all those who conduct business with the organization—and to the public at large with whom you are building trust.
- **Encourage ongoing disclosure.** One way to deter board members from hiding or ignoring conflicts of interest is to require ongoing disclosure. Most organizations query potential board members about conflicts during the selection process. But you can take this effort one step further by ensuring that board members understand that they are responsible for disclosing

new and emerging conflicts throughout their tenure.

Although healthcare organizations may ask board members to periodically update their conflict-of-interest statements, ultimately each individual is responsible for disclosing such information as soon as questions arise.

- **Create a board culture.** Several decades ago, author Robert Greenleaf urged healthcare executives to guide their organizations by adopting a "servant leadership" mentality—a concept that can be applied to your board. By instilling this culture, you may prevent conflicts of interest before they arise. Directors on the board of a healthcare organization—be it for-profit or not-for-profit—are there to serve the organization. If the culture of the board reflects the servant leadership philosophy, it will be easier for individuals to deal with conflicts because they will put the welfare of the organization first.

- **Assign directors to appropriate committees.** Since most board work is done within a committee structure, steer members away from committees with tasks that will likely collide with their personal interests. This brings us to your first question regarding the necessity of severing all business relationships. If a banker from a small town is on the community hospital's board of directors and the hospital is conducting business with that bank, the banker should not be a member of the finance committee. Rather, he or she could better serve the hospital in another capacity, perhaps on the quality assurance committee. Of course, when business that causes a conflict of interest is brought before the board in its entirety, the individual for whom the conflict arises can always leave the board room during discussion and should always abstain from voting. However, if a board member is a partner in a consulting firm that is attempting to enter into a major consulting contract with the hospital, it is best for the organization to avoid using that consulting firm.

While the steps described above may act as deterrents, to believe that healthcare organizations can avoid all conflicts of interest is naive. Following are several actions that can be used to address violations of disclosure:

- **Use an independent review.** Once conflicts of interest are disclosed by directors, the board faces the sticky question of what to do about the situation. Allowing the rest of the board to decide how to address the conflict could be problematic. In the context of resolving the conflict, you may run the risk of arousing a new set of conflicts for other members of the board. Thus, an independent review from an in-house legal staff or an outside legal counsel may be more prudent.
- **Suggest resignation.** If the conflict cannot be resolved, the individual should resign from the board. He or she can serve in the healthcare organization in another capacity, but not in a policy-making position.

In addition to conflicts of interest between individual board members and the hospitals they serve, other situations may arise between the hospital and the community itself that the board will need to address. In the smaller communities you mention in your question, for example, boards may need to address the business relationships they have in town vs. those they have outside of town. If a small community has one bank and one hospital, will the hospital conduct business with that bank exclusively to show its support for the community? The conflict here—regardless of whether a banker is on the hospital board—is between the fiduciary responsibility of the board to the hospital and its responsibility to stimulate the local community and its business. If the bank cannot be competitive in its offerings, the board might carve out a part of the healthcare organization's business for the bank to service, thus strengthening that bank and supporting the community.

While we cannot address every conflict-of-interest scenario in this forum, two important guidelines can help you deal with such situations appropriately: The board needs to conduct very open and honest discussions among its members, and the board should be prepared to explain or defend its position just as openly to the community. With these two goals in mind, you will usually make a decision that is in the best interest of your organization.

January/February 2003

Evaluating Claims of Conscience

William A. Nelson, PhD, and Cedric K. Dark, MD, MPH

Several physicians at my facility have been citing the conscience clause to opt out of providing certain treatments. How can I be certain that their claims of conscience are sincere and thus warrant honoring?

Before attempting to evaluate a claim of conscience, we must first understand the ethical nature of conscience clauses. In addition, since these clauses vary legally from state to state, be sure to research the legislation as it applies to you and your organization. Several important considerations to take into account include:

- Who is eligible to use the conscience clause?
- What procedures are covered by the conscience clause?
- What principles might an individual who wishes to use the conscience clause cite?

In general terms, conscience clauses protect the ethical right of physicians and others involved in patient care to object to performing a particular treatment on the basis of their moral and/or religious views. Often, the types of treatment providers can refuse are limited to reproductive health or end-of-life issues (e.g., abortion, sterilization, physician-assisted suicide). Although most conscience clauses require that claims are grounded in religious or moral views, in some jurisdictions claims may be based upon personal judgment or philosophical views.

The responsibility for evaluating claims of conscience should be dispersed across several levels of leadership. Initially, a claim of conscience should be brought to the petitioner's immediate supervisor—a head nurse, attending physician, etc. At this stage, the supervisor has the duty to evaluate the validity of the claim. Valid claims should be based on moral or religious (and possibly cultural) beliefs about a medically reasonable and available procedure or treatment. However, the objection cannot be based on personal interest, stated public and/or hospital policy, medical opinion, convenience, prejudice, or arbitrariness.

Situations that fail to adhere to these general standards should not be considered valid uses of the conscience clause. Claims that are, however, deemed valid according to the above criteria may pass to the next level: a review board composed of members from various ethnic, religious, and academic settings. Optimally, this panel should represent the diversified demographics within your healthcare organization so that all staff might find an advocate. The mission of the review board is to determine whether valid claims of conscience are indeed genuine claims. Genuineness can be established whenever

- the objection fits within a coherent system of moral, religious, cultural, or philosophical beliefs,
- this belief reflects a consistently and diligently held core value of the petitioner,
- the belief is such a key component of the petitioner's internal framework that violation of that belief would cause significant harm to him or her, or
- it would be inconsistent with the petitioner's core values to participate in the procedure or treatment.

In the instance that the request is not determined to be genuine and hence subsequently denied, a mechanism for appeal (perhaps even to a court of appropriate jurisdiction) should exist. But whenever the review process finds the conscientious objection both valid and genuine, your organization should seek a solution. In order to reasonably accommodate the valid request, healthcare executives must ensure that no undue hardship falls upon the organization, its employees, or the patient. The following organizational conditions must be satisfied before implementing an appeal of provider conscience:

- The quality of patient care must not be sacrificed (nonabandonment).
- An alternate provider should be found who is willing and competent to perform the procedure or treatment.
- An undue burden should not fall on other employees.
- The responsibility from which the petitioner seeks to be exempted should not be a fundamental element of his or her job or profession.

As long as these criteria can be satisfied, the healthcare organization should not hesitate to accept and implement the petitioner's claim of conscience. If, however, any of these criteria cannot be satisfied, a reassignment or possibly termination of the petitioner's employment may be necessary. As stated earlier, an appeals process (possibly external) should exist in the event that reassignment or termination results. The response to each case should be recorded and referred to whenever future cases arise. Similar to other organizational procedures, the process should be assessed to ensure it is effectively fulfilling its purpose.

Following these guidelines, you should be able to institute a program that will enable you to foster an ethical organization by respecting the conscience of your providers while continuing to deliver high-quality healthcare.

March/April 2003

Revealing Inconvenient Truths

Paul B. Hofmann, DrPH, FACHE

My organization has a tendency not to disclose negative financial results or other unfavorable information in a timely manner. Since this propensity seems to be part of our organizational culture, how can it be changed?

The likelihood of a delay is usually a reflection of one or more factors: the news itself, the person responsible for communicating the information, and the organizational culture. The bad news can be no one's "fault," yet the lower the person's status within the organization, the more likely that individual may fear being blamed. On occasion, the CEO may be the one not receiving full disclosure by the chief financial officer or another senior executive. Nonetheless, the harsh facts may be of such magnitude that withholding them could jeopardize the organization's ability to implement corrective measures.

No one actually enjoys communicating bad news, so there is an understandable inclination to withhold, delay, or minimize such news. In some instances, a manager may provide only partial data, omitting adverse elements or critical interpretations. At least in the short term, both the report's author and recipients are spared the anticipated discomfort associated with releasing and receiving unpleasant information. The manager may even rationalize that limited disclosure or nondisclosure is not really deceptive, or even if he or she concedes this possibility, it is regarded as benign deception. Another common rationalization is that others do not really need to know about a negative outcome.

There is irrefutable proof that disclosure of medical errors is indispensable in preventing and reducing subsequent errors, but management mistakes also occur. Concealing them is both unethical and counterproductive. One of the keys is to promote an organizational culture that not only permits but also explicitly encourages full and timely disclosure.

If your organization historically has condoned withholding, delaying, minimizing, or misrepresenting negative financial results, it is likely the problem is not restricted to fiscal issues. The following 10 steps should be considered to change a generic predilection to hide inconvenient truths:

1.   Revisit the organization's values statement to ensure that the timely communication of pertinent information, both positive and negative, is underscored. Then, the reality must match the rhetoric.

2.   Suggest this topic be placed on the agenda of a board, management, and/or department-head retreat. Candid discussion can reinforce a genuine commitment to being consistently honest and timely in all communications.

3.   Recognize managers for conveying adverse results in a timely and constructive way, and counsel those who do not. Although these situations should occur infrequently, such actions will show that management is serious about this issue.

4.   Discourage the development and distribution of overly optimistic reports intended to generate support for new projects, programs, or services. When the justification is so compelling that it borders on hyperbole, expectations will likely fall short, and the validity of future proposals will be suspect.

5.   Be aware that the level of knowledge about healthcare economics varies widely throughout an organization, and do

not presume that everyone understands routinely distributed reports or the current reimbursement environment. For instance, do board members really understand what is meant by "contractual allowances"? After assessing what people know and believe, you can design programs to address gaps, resulting in better-informed constituencies who are more capable of interpreting adverse developments.

6. Develop and distribute comparative information that can place the organization's position in context. Be sure to note whether negative trends are affecting your organization alone, as compared with the entire field or geographic area.

7. Prepare contingency plans in anticipation that negative financial conditions will require some painful measures. Denial can be a powerful deterrent to confronting economic downturns, and a reluctance to solicit and coordinate plans almost always ensures a less timely response.

8. Determine in advance who might misuse or exploit negative information (perhaps disgruntled members of the board, medical staff, media, or union), and develop a strategy for each group that emphasizes education and full disclosure to establish and maintain credibility. When accompanied by practical remedies to address the problem, this approach should foster respect for management.

9. Act promptly when a negative situation is the result of clear incompetence or malfeasance. Procrastination or other forms of avoidance will only exacerbate the problem and further undermine the organization's reputation.

10. Identify a few colleagues who can be trusted to offer sound recommendations, not just advice they think you want to hear during a serious crisis. Even the most capable managers make errors in judgment, and it is helpful to have access to individuals who will thoughtfully challenge your thinking.

Wanting to avoid the emotional pain associated with revealing inconvenient truths is a natural preference, but personal as well as organizational integrity and credibility are at stake. Furthermore, a culture that promotes the timely release of negative information on a consistent basis should discourage tendencies to cover up or misrepresent bad news. At a time when the public's confidence in corporate management has deteriorated for well-publicized reasons, healthcare organizations should take every opportunity to promote full disclosure.

September/October 2003

Compliance and Ethics: A Critical Interdependence

Rich Cohan , FACHE

What is the difference between ethical and compliant behavior? As a senior leader in my organization, what are my personal responsibilities to foster a culture that encourages both types of behavior?

"No man is an island entire of itself; every man is a piece of the Continent, a part of the main," said the famous British poet John Donne. While this statement speaks to the role of the individual in society, it also describes the way senior-level healthcare executives must view their behavior in the context of their organizations. In short, what each of us as leaders does is directly transferable to our stakeholders (patients, employees, physicians, and volunteers) and the ethical culture within the organization. Following are several steps healthcare leaders can take to foster an environment that is not only compliant but also ethical.

STEP 1: IDENTIFY THE DIFFERENCE BETWEEN COMPLIANCE AND ETHICS

Quite often, the terms "compliant" and "ethical" behavior are mistakenly used interchangeably when they are actually distinct concepts.

Compliant behavior means that you, your organization, and your employees obey the myriad laws, rules, and regulations you must follow to operate your healthcare business in the context of other healthcare businesses in your state and/or across the country. Important? Absolutely. Compliant behavior reduces the risk of costly litigation, bad press, and a loss of stock value for public entities. Ethical conduct takes an organization to the next level—a level at which decisions are made not only to comply with the law, but furthermore, to always do the right thing. Doing the right thing sounds simplistic, but just what does it mean? It means, for example, that a hospital CEO and board of trustees decide to maintain a department that is losing a significant amount of money because the department's patients and the entire community would not have the services they need should the unit be closed.

In the end, as a leader, understanding the relationship that exists between acting in a compliant manner and leading with ethical commitment is of paramount importance in how you are perceived by your stakeholders and what the organization's ethical climate is. It means being a champion not only for doing things right (compliance) but even more importantly, doing the right things (compliance plus ethics).

STEP 2: IDENTIFY YOUR MISSION, VALUES, AND CORPORATE RESPONSIBILITY

In healthcare organizations, a climate that is both compliant and ethical starts with and will be driven by the mission, values, and visible dedication to corporate responsibility. In this context, corporate responsibility is the confluence of ethics, compliance, and commitment to our communities and the environment. Our mission statement tells who we are, what we do, whom we serve, and what is unique about our organization. Our values statements, on the other hand, tend to be much more personal. In many instances, they contain single-word concepts like integrity, quality, respect, or diversity.

The key point is that the mission and values of an organization are continually seen by stakeholders within our facilities, in our codes of conduct, on our Web pages, and through countless other forums. Mission and values help set the compliance and ethical tone by the words or concepts chosen, as well as by those that are not included. After all, how often do we see the phrase "law abiding" in our values statements? The connotation, I would argue, is too negative to send the message we want to convey to our employees and other stakeholders. On the other hand, "integrity" is an all-encompassing word. One definition is "the quality or state of being of sound moral principle; uprightness, honesty, and sincerity." Creating a culture based on integrity, then, marries compliance to ethics.

STEP 3: MEASURE THE CURRENT ETHICAL ENVIRONMENT

As leaders in our organizations, we must understand that to establish an ethical climate means that we must first understand what the current environment is. A good compliance program will always include monitoring and auditing as a key component. One way to move from a one-dimensional, compliance-focused environment to a more complex ethical plane is to measure the organization's current environment. Using an ethics audit, this process can begin with a survey designed to help leaders understand how their stakeholders perceive ethics in the organization. This survey can serve many purposes. First, it provides objective data that can be benchmarked against other organizations. Second, and more importantly, the audit offers a glimpse at the ethical issues that are most important to your stakeholders. ACHE offers an Ethics Self-Assessment—located in the About ACHE area of www.ache.org—that can help individuals identify areas for improvement and further reflection.

A formalized audit is just one of many measurement tools. Less formal methods can also sufficiently assess the ethical climate of the organization. Focus groups, team meetings, and even rumors can provide valuable insight into how leaders' decisions are being perceived. Just be sure to have a process in place that captures feedback and includes a mechanism for acting on what you learn.

STEP 4: ACT ON RESULTS

Taking action based on audit activities is the next step. Once a concern is identified, senior leaders can determine the best course of action. In a compliance context, this action might include involving an attorney, paying money to a federal health program, and/or disciplining employees. In an ethical context, actions may include creating an efficient communication path that allows stakeholders to share issues, concerns, and solutions. Internal newsletters, department meetings, employee forums, and an organization's intranet can help disseminate information. Using case studies to train leaders can help the organization's leaders work through a variety of issues that might not have clear-cut answers. The ensuing discussions will provide valuable insight into a given leader's ethical decision-making process.

STEP 5: BE AWARE OF YOUR VISIBILITY

As the quote in the beginning of this article states, we are all "a part of the main." This statement illuminates the reason perceptions of others so significantly affect the organization's ethical climate—and why senior leaders play an important role in fostering it. One word: Visibility! From a compliance perspective, each leader is a self-motivated, autonomous individual doing things right to keep the organization and themselves out of trouble. While this is all well and good, healthcare leaders are very visible, often acting as a spokesperson for their department, their division, their hospital, or their system.

But their visibility carries over further. For example, let's say the CEO and members of the executive team of a community hospital are seen dining together recently and repeatedly in the finest establishments with several of the leading surgeons from the key surgical practice in the area. The group is also noted to have played golf the following weekend—and the surgeons all have towels and balls with the hospital's name on them.

A month later, the hospital announces that it is going to be renovating a number of the OR suites used by this surgical group. A number of stakeholders know that this was not in the capital budget, and rumor has it that the equipment being replaced was really not that old. As a matter of fact, the OR director, who is normally a quiet person, has become vocal in his displeasure with the decision.

While the leaders of this hospital may talk a good game, rumor and innuendo can arise from many places and can do significant damage to the ethical climate of the organization—even if they were acting in compliance with the laws and regulations that govern their organization. But if a key value of this organization is honesty or integrity, the CEO and the executive team must be held, and hold themselves, to a higher level of responsibility beyond mere compliant behavior to the higher purpose of moral principles, a.k.a. ethics.

January/February 2004

Beyond HIPAA: Ethics in the e-Health Arena

John Mack

As the area of online, interactive healthcare communications continues to expand, healthcare organizations must be concerned about securing individual privacy and fostering strong ethical behavior. What are the ethical principles relevant to e-health? How should healthcare organizations develop and promote ethics guidelines and codes of conduct for websites and electronic patient information?

The American healthcare system is undergoing a reform in which technology—and especially the Internet—is playing a major role. While HIPAA's privacy and security rules have paved the way for e-health applications by easing some concerns about patient privacy and the security of electronic health information, HIPAA offers a floor, rather than a ceiling, for health privacy. The legislation does not apply to health information and services offered through the Internet by nonhealthcare professionals, and it is silent on other extralegal ramifications of e-health, such as the quality of health information online and the biases that may be introduced by the commercialization of e-health. These issues must be addressed to build trust in e-health and ensure its success.

THE GOAL: BUILD TRUST

Trust is fundamental to healthcare. Patients rely on healthcare providers to keep their personal information confidential, to provide accurate and appropriate information about their conditions and possible treatments, and to recommend the therapy they believe to be in the patient's best interest.

But trust can be particularly difficult to achieve in the anonymous, virtual environment of the Internet where anyone who has access to a computer, an online connection, and modest technical skill is able to set up a website offering health information, products, or services, regardless of his or her qualifications. Trust was especially in short supply during the heyday of the Internet "dot-com boom" era (1995 through 2000) when many entrepreneurs established commercial, for-profit health information websites. This early phase of the Internet was likened to the Wild West—a land without formal laws in which you ventured at your peril. It was left up to consumers themselves to determine what they were dealing with.

THE E-HEALTH CODE OF ETHICS

In response to ever-growing public scrutiny of the Internet health arena, several organizations have championed e-health ethics initiatives. These include

- Health On the Net (HON), *Code of Conduct* (www.hon.ch/HONcode/Conduct.html);
- American Medical Association, *Guidelines for Medical and Health Information Sites on the Internet*;
- Health Internet Ethics (Hi-Ethics), *Ethical Principles for Offering Internet Health Services to Consumers* (www.hiethics.org/Principles/index.asp);

- Internet Healthcare Coalition, *e-Health Code of Ethics* (www.ihealthcoalition.org/ethics/ethics.html); and
- URAC, "Health Web Site Standards" (www.urac.org/documents/HealthWebSitev1-0Standards040122.pdf).

The goals of these initiatives and organizations are to draft ethical guidelines for creating credible and trustworthy health information and services on the Internet. There has been much cross-fertilization among these groups in terms of shared members and documents. The resulting guidelines, codes, and standards, therefore, share much in common.

The *e-Health Code of Ethics,* developed by the nonprofit, non-aligned Internet Healthcare Coalition, was created by the largest and most diverse group of stakeholders, including members of all the organizations mentioned above. The coalition based its initiative and the resulting *e-Health Code of Ethics* on collaboration and consensus among a broad mix of stakeholders, including traditional healthcare organizations, commercial Internet health information publishers, regulatory organizations, and most important, individual consumers. The coalition's *e-Health Code of Ethics* aims to help healthcare managers and executives operationalize e-health ethical leadership within their organizations. The code provides what I call the "eight commandments" of e-health ethics. As such, it offers the moral and ethical framework

---

e-Health Code of Ethics: An Executive Summary

Candor: Disclose information that, if known by consumers, would likely affect their understanding or use of the site, or purchase or use of a product or service.

Honesty: Be truthful and not deceptive.

Quality: Provide health information that is accurate, easy to understand, and up to date. Provide the information users need to make their own

---

(Continued on following page)

judgments about the health information, products, or services provided by the site.

Informed Consent: Respect users' right to determine whether or how their personal data may be collected, used, or shared.

Privacy: Respect the obligation to protect users' privacy.

Professionalism in Online Healthcare: Respect fundamental ethical obligations to patients and clients. Inform and educate patients and clients about the limitations of online healthcare.

Responsible Partnering: Ensure that organizations and sites with which they affiliate are trustworthy.

Accountability: Provide meaningful opportunity for users to give feedback to the site.

that other groups can interpret to satisfy the individual, practical needs of different kinds of stakeholders (see box).

TIPS FOR E-HEALTH DEVELOPERS AND EXECUTIVES

Healthcare executives at the highest levels can ensure that proper ethical standards are adopted to govern their e-health applications by keeping the following in mind:

- Remember that adopting any of the codes mentioned above is a step forward from no code at all. All of the codes contain sound advice on how to conduct business on the Internet. It is critical that healthcare executives educate consumers about ethical practices and how to distinguish e-health services based on ethical principles from those that are not.
- Website developers and e-health executives should practice "ethical due diligence" with regard to choosing their business partners and sites to which they link. Your trusted reputation

is often transferred to your partners. Don't let this trust be betrayed by partners who do not comply with the same high ethical standards that you do.

- It is important to train key employees in ethical standards. Often, mistakes are made by well-intentioned employees who are ignorant of the issues and who do not know how to identify and resolve ethical dilemmas. Ensure that key employees and managers are familiar with the ethical issues for creating trustworthy health sites.
- For now, adopting an ethics code is voluntary. Organizations that adopt a code should perform a critical self-assessment of their websites to ensure they comply with the code. Participating in URAC's fee-based Web Site Accreditation program may help you formalize this process and identify critical gaps between ethical standards and actual practice.
- If you do adopt a code, be sure to promote it to consumers and patients who use your e-health services. This can be a competitive advantage, but more important, you can use the code to teach users how to find credible health information and services through other websites they are likely to visit.

Meeting the e-health challenges ahead calls for innovative management and a new focus on ethical issues. Healthcare providers, payers, and consumers share a responsibility to ensure the value and integrity of e-health by exercising judgment in creating and using the technology according to the highest possible ethical standards.

September/October 2004

Accepting Vendor Gifts

Jeffrey C. Oak, PhD

Many suppliers and vendors provide gifts to people throughout our hospital, ranging from lavish lunches to tickets to premier events. To attract and retain physicians, our administrators often do the same for our doctors. Can you provide guidelines that can help us draw the line between what is appropriate and what may be a conflict of interest?

The receiving and giving of gifts is one of the more ethically sensitive issues in healthcare, and you are wise to take an "ethics pause" to carefully consider where and how to draw meaningful lines. On the one hand, we are social beings, and the giving and receiving of gifts is a common practice that can smooth the sometimes hard edges of social interaction. Moreover, the foundation of any business is a network of relationships that are fostered through kindnesses, courtesies, and the giving and receiving of gifts. On the other hand, practices that may be acceptable and entirely appropriate in certain business relationships outside healthcare may be ethically problematic—and even illegal—in the healthcare domain.

It may help to clarify some legal issues before examining more deeply the ethical issues at the heart of gift giving and receiving.

LEGAL ISSUES

The giving of gifts is one of the principal areas that can trigger what are commonly called the "referral statutes," otherwise known as the antikickback and Stark II laws.

The antikickback criminal statute prohibits the exchange of anything of value where one—even secondary—purpose of the exchange is to induce or reward business referrals for any item or service that may be reimbursed, even partly, by a federal healthcare program such as Medicare or Medicaid. The statute identifies a series of "safe harbors"; if the particular facts and circumstances fit squarely within these harbors, the statute is not triggered. But each safe harbor has exacting requirements, and there is little room for error.

In addition to antikickback, the other referral statute that can be triggered by the giving and receiving of gifts is Stark II. Stark II prohibits hospitals and other providers from submitting any claim for payment by any payer—public or private—if that claim is the result of a referral by a physician (or immediate family member) with whom the hospital has a prohibited financial relationship. The list of prohibited financial relationships is long and covers a broad range of direct and indirect ownership or compensation, including

- stock ownership;
- partnership interest;
- secured debt;
- rental or personal services contracts;
- salary, recruitment incentives, and income guarantees; and
- gifts and gratuities.

In short, gifts in the healthcare setting can easily run afoul of either the antikickback or Stark II laws.

ETHICAL ISSUES

There are also potential ethical issues that can arise as a result of receiving gifts or other things of value. Exploring these ethical issues can help us understand the deeper logic at play and assist in the development of meaningful guidelines.

One of the basic ethical assumptions in the practice of medicine is that clinical decision making will be independent, objective, and focused first and foremost on the best interests of the patient. There are many who stand in various places in the long chain of clinical decision making: physicians who provide direct care to patients, hospital-based physicians (e.g., anesthesiologists, radiologists, pathologists), nurses, pharmacists, and those in the supply chain. If any of these decision makers receives a gift as an inducement or reward for certain kinds of referrals, that gift has the potential to make clinical decision making be—or appear to be—less than fully independent and objective. It can encourage overutilization or inappropriate utilization. And it can even introduce patient safety and quality-of-care risks.

Another basic assumption of medicine is that decision making will take into account the proper stewardship of public resources and public funds. In addition to the risks to patient care, gifts have the potential to increase costs to federal healthcare programs, beneficiaries, or enrollees, thus compromising public trust in the healthcare enterprise.

GUIDELINES

At the heart of giving and receiving gifts is the importance of avoiding conflicts of interest. A conflict of interest exists whenever the loyalty of an individual is divided between his or her official responsibilities and an outside interest such as a gift or other thing of value. A good rule to follow is that a potential conflict of interest exists any time an objective observer of our actions might wonder if these actions are motivated by something other than our official responsibilities to the care of patients and the proper stewardship of public resources. When it comes to conflicts of interest, appearances matter. Even if decision making is not actually influenced by a gift, the fact that it could *appear* to be influenced by that gift is itself a problem. Following are some additional guidelines to help you ensure appropriate giving and receiving of gifts.

- **Understand that the fact your golf partner can do it doesn't mean you can.** Gift-giving practices that may be perfectly acceptable in other industries may not be ethically acceptable— or legal—in healthcare.
- **Educate, educate, educate.** Codify your policy on gift giving and receiving, and then educate the staff. Start with the board, then move to senior executives, medical staff, managers, and supervisors.
- **Set dollar limits cautiously.** If you set a dollar limit—and many organizations do—be sure that all senior leaders are prepared to enforce it *and* live by it. And be sure to state whether it is a onetime limit or cumulative (e.g., one-year period).
- **Trust and verify.** Trust your people to do the right thing. Then find meaningful ways to verify that they do.
- **Provide an escape hatch.** Inevitably, employees will find themselves in a situation where they feel they cannot refuse an impermissible gift. Anticipate this and provide an escape hatch in the form of a "script" for what to say and a process to follow if the script doesn't work. For example, employees can be trained that if all else fails, they should accept the gift, notify management, make arrangements to donate it to an appropriate charity, and document what happened.
- **Ask to see the vendor's code of ethics, then insist that they follow it.** The pharmaceutical industry, for example, has a code that provides detailed guidance on what gifts are ethically permissible for salespeople to give to providers. Watch to see if

vendors follow their own rules, and you'll quickly be able to make judgments about their ethics.

- **Draw the lines, then keep your distance from them.** A classic *New Yorker* cartoon pictures a pin-striped executive who says to his managers, "We've got to draw a line on ethical behavior . . . and then get as close to that line as possible." Don't follow this example! Appearances count, and from the viewpoint of others, being close to an ethical line can look like you've crossed it.

Most important, try to remain as objective as possible. Imagine what is going on in your organization as a kind of theatrical production. Assume the position of the neutral observer, and try to assess how the critics would evaluate what is happening on stage. When viewed in this manner, lavish lunches or tickets to expensive events may certainly appear inappropriate.

July/August 2005

Ethical Implications
of Transparency

William A. Nelson, PhD, and Justin Campfield

How does transparency enhance healthcare, and when is it ethically appropriate to withhold information regarding a hospital or health system?

A great deal has been written about the importance of organizational transparency in healthcare. Transparency—an open, honest and accessible approach to the communication of information with patients, employees and the community—is a widely accepted ideal, but the extent of organizational transparency varies dramatically from facility to facility.

Transparency should be the standard of behavior for a healthcare organization and should pervade its culture on all levels. Situations related to disclosure typically fall under three relationship arenas: patient-caregiver, employee-employer, and organization-community relationships. However, occasions may arise when withholding information is morally justified.

Truthful and full disclosure of healthcare-related information is fundamental to a patient-caregiver relationship. Failure to do so undermines the integrity of the shared decision-making process. The extent to which honesty and openness in the patient-caregiver relationship have been tested recently includes whether medical errors should be disclosed to patients or families. Many have argued that adverse events should not be disclosed because of the potential for increased litigation. Others have taken the position that disclosure is required despite the arguable litigation concern because truthfulness should be the norm in all patient communication and the provider's organization. This line of reasoning has led some healthcare organizations, including the Department of Veterans Affairs, to draft and implement a national policy requiring truthful disclosure following an adverse event.

A good employee-employer relationship requires honest and open communication. Transparency of information about the organization's practices, decisions and expectations of each employee can enhance employee morale and commitment to the organization. For example, hospitals and health systems that proactively develop and propagate ethical practice guidelines for recurring employee conflicts can prevent ethical uncertainty and distress, a leading cause of employee burnout.

The same line of moral reasoning that has led employers and caregivers to accept the value and importance of disclosure of information also is appropriate for healthcare organizations and their leaders in relationship to the community they serve. Failing to be open and honest about the organization and its practices can be harmful to the organization and undermine its image. Not only is transparency morally correct but it makes sense from a business perspective. A patient's perception of an organization as being honest and truthful will influence the decision of where to seek care and affect overall satisfaction with the organization. Transparency can enhance the organization's credibility, the public's trust and the community's commitment to the healthcare organization.

In addition to sharing basic information about the organization through means such as its website, transparency ideally should include

- the organization's mission, objectives, and values;
- a description of the scope of services and staff;
- patient care and disease-related information;

- quality measures and reports; and
- healthcare-related pricing.

Despite the moral basis for transparency in all relationships, situations may arise in which withholding information from the community is morally justifiable. As is the case with all moral principles, they are not absolute. However, because violating any moral principle, including truth telling and open communication, is a significant action, valid justification for the withholding of information is required.

The violation of the moral principle is based on a clear assessment that the disclosure would cause greater harm than the potential benefit. Some examples where it may be morally acceptable to limit transparency regarding community-organization relationships include patient health and personal information; employee personnel information, such as salaries; and proprietary information, such as expansion plans, the hospital's strategic plan (including new, expanded or prioritized service lines) and negotiations with insurance companies. Patient and employee information can be morally justified for nondisclosure because of the need to protect the patient's and employee's privacy. An exception may include those occasions when the law requires the reporting of specific unlawful behaviors by a patient or employee. Withholding proprietary information also is justified to protect an organization's financial security and ability to remain competitive in the marketplace.

Fortunately for healthcare executives, when it comes to decision making regarding whether or not to disclose certain information, they are not alone. In situations of uncertainty, healthcare executives should seek the advice and counsel of the facility's ethics committee, legal counsel, public relations professional and possibly a community representative *before, during,* and *after* a transparency decision is made. Each can contribute to the decision-making process, and all should aim to foster the organization's mission and values of doing the right thing for the patients served.

Even after a decision to either disclose or not disclose information has been made, work still needs to be done. Healthcare executives may consider turning to their public relations professionals to facilitate the decision with an appropriate communications strategy. A communications plan for *not* communicating something may seem counterintuitive, but as with any major decision, many stakeholders, such as physicians, employees, and board members, are privy to information involving transparency decisions. Public relations professionals can be counted on to communicate the nondisclosure decision, and the process used to determine it, to all appropriate parties. Often making sure key stakeholders are well informed can prevent an internal issue from being debated in the public forum.

November/December 2006

Should Hospitals Always Bill for Costs?

Paul B. Hofmann, DrPH, FACHE

Occasionally, during surgery, an expensive surgical implant has to be discarded because it cannot be returned to the supplier after an unsuccessful attempt to place it in the patient, usually because it is the wrong size. What should we do? Bill full charges, bill only for the cost of the implant or not bill at all?

In dealing with this type of dilemma with ethical dimensions, it is frequently helpful to consider five fundamental questions:

1. What are the relevant ethical facts?
2. What additional information is needed?
3. What are the ethical/value conflicts?
4. What is the most appropriate response after considering alternatives?
5. What is the ethical basis for your decision?

Addressing these questions increases the likelihood that the review process will be thorough and thoughtful. If a small group is appointed to conduct this process, legitimate differences in opinion may occur. But careful deliberation should generate more creative analysis, observations and options than having only one person undertake the task.

WHAT ARE THE RELEVANT ETHICAL FACTS?

The facts appear to be self-evident. The hospital incurred the cost of the implant and it cannot be used for another patient or returned to the supplier. Also, if payment is not received from the patient/insurance carrier, the unreimbursed cost will essentially be subsidized by all patients. Evidently, this problem has occurred in the past and will probably happen again.

WHAT ADDITIONAL INFORMATION IS NEEDED?

Too often, there is a tendency to "rush to judgment" and to conclude prematurely that the answer to a particular dilemma is obvious. One of the advantages of engaging several people in examining such a case is a more robust assessment of not only what is known but also what additional facts could be helpful.

Among the questions you should raise are the following:

- Is there an existing policy that may cover this type of situation?
- How frequent is the problem?
- Has there been a change in the frequency with which the problem has occurred?
- What types of implants are involved? What is the monthly or annual amount of unreimbursed costs for each kind?
- Is there any discernable pattern? For example, do one or two orthopedic surgeons account for most of the cases?
- If the problem is more common among some physicians or procedures than others, what steps can be taken to identify and implement best practices?
- In addition to financial and ethical factors, what legal and public relation aspects should be evaluated?
- Is the problem more significant here in comparison to similar hospitals?
- How do other hospitals deal with this issue?

- Is it recognized as a problem from the payers' or suppliers' perspective?
- Would it be worthwhile to arrange a discussion with two or three suppliers to engage them in contributing to a solution?

WHAT ARE THE ETHICAL/VALUE CONFLICTS?

The principal conflicts revolve around fairness, honesty, justice, stewardship, and promise-keeping; resolving them requires raising yet more questions: Is it fair to charge a patient for an implant that was not used? If a charge is processed, how should the charge be represented on the patient's billing statement? Should the dollar amount comprise only the cost of the implant or should the amount include a conventional mark up? If the patient is not billed, is there an acceptable alternative for obtaining payment? Given a fiduciary responsibility to manage the hospital's limited resources effectively, what are the implications of simply absorbing the costs? How will the hospital fulfill its formally stated commitment to relate charges to actual costs?

WHAT IS THE APPROPRIATE RESPONSE AFTER CONSIDERING ALTERNATIVES?

The decision will largely depend on the answers obtained from the factual and ethical questions posed above. Because the issue cannot simply be ignored, a sound and defensible policy should be developed. Assuming every step was taken to minimize the number of unusable implants, including the correction of any quality of care issues—and that the problem is limited to specific surgical procedures—adjusting the implant charge for these procedures to cover the projected cost of the unused implants is one solution.

WHAT IS THE ETHICAL BASIS FOR YOUR DECISION?

The costs incurred for unusable implants and other medical devices should be recovered, but it would be unfair to spread these costs across all surgical and nonsurgical patients. Only patients who receive implants should bear the incremental expense based on the presumption they are at potential risk for not having the correct-sized implant. But prior to implementation, the hospital's ethics committee should review a draft policy that provides the full ethical and financial rationale.

FINAL COMMENTS

In 2001, Bradley Googins, of the Center for Corporate Citizenship at Boston College, said, "Good corporate citizenship is fiscal transparency, the demonstration of a corporate social conscience and evidence that corporate values are more than pretty words on a framed plaque." If these values are more than rhetoric, organizational integrity requires constant vigilance to prevent business errors of omission and commission.

The movement toward greater disclosure and transparency of hospital charges is rapidly accelerating. In the absence of thoughtful and clear policies, arbitrary and inconsistent billing practices are inevitable. Only by conducting a comprehensive audit and asking the right questions can an organization identify problems, produce solutions and avoid the potential financial, legal and ethical costs of inappropriate practices.

July/August 2007

Ethical Issues and Disaster Planning

Paul B. Hofmann, DrPH, FACHE

Every healthcare organization is obligated to maintain an effective disaster plan. Triage is only one obvious component with significant ethical dimensions. How should this component, as well as others with ethical implications, be addressed?

Although disaster planning and drills are obligatory, these activities are seldom approached with enthusiasm because most people would prefer not to think about the prospect of having to confront the potentially devastating consequences of a natural disaster, terrorist attack, or pandemic. Nonetheless, anticipating the need to make difficult decisions in times of crisis is imperative if these decisions are going to be both effective and ethically sound.

PERFORMING TRIAGE AND REVERSE TRIAGE

In the article "Lifeboat Ethics: Considerations in the Discharge of Inpatients for the Creation of Hospital Surge Capacity," Kraus, Levy, and Kelen say that if hospitals and their staff are still able to function in an overwhelming disaster, the organizations should be considered lifeboats with insufficient capacity to take care of everyone. Therefore, decisions must be made about who will best be served. In the article, published in the journal *Disaster Medicine and Public Health Preparedness* (June 2007), the authors recommend that an objective appraisal be made not only of prospective patients but also inpatients whose needs may be less acute than others requiring treatment.

Such situations demand advance planning. Individuals should consider how various ethical principles will be followed, such as respecting an individual's right of self-determination, maximizing benefit, avoiding harm, distributing benefits fairly, promisekeeping, fidelity, and truth-telling. Not all these principles and the values associated with them can be accommodated all the time. Organizations must ask themselves: How will conflicts be reconciled and a proper balance be maintained? At least part of the answer to that question should be found in the organization's vision, mission, and value statements.

EDUCATING THE PUBLIC AND MANAGING EXPECTATIONS

As evident during and after Hurricane Katrina, neither hospitals nor the public knew what to do or how to deal with this unprecedented disaster. There was an illusion that the healthcare system and its institutional providers would always be available and capable of responding to the public's need for vital services. No one was prepared to deal with the impact of inoperable hospitals.

A hospital's disaster program must have a contingency plan that recognizes the possibility it will be unable to function in whole or in part at its current location. Once these possibilities are addressed, then all the hospital's stakeholders must be educated about well-designed alternatives.

PRACTICING EVIDENCE-BASED DISASTER MEDICINE

Physicians and nurses who have worked in disaster conditions emphasize that there is a discrepancy between the theoretical aspects of disaster planning and the harsh reality of contending with an actual disaster. They do not discount the importance of conducting drills, but they assert that drills "are generally not authentic" despite planners' best efforts.

In regard to disaster planning, there is a common disconnect between what health professionals know is appropriate and their behavior. For example, do we and our staff have disaster kits at home? How can this lack of experience and complacency be overcome to increase the level of preparedness for real catastrophes that affect our institutions?

Healthcare executives have a moral imperative to plan and prepare well. The haunting images and descriptions of disasters in the United States and abroad are often quickly forgotten. However, by reviewing calamities and the vivid insights and lessons conveyed by disaster specialists, healthcare professionals can raise the level of familiarity with evidence-based disaster medicine.

MEETING THE NEEDS OF CAREGIVERS AND THEIR FAMILIES

Before reporting to work during a disaster, people can be expected to take care of themselves and their families first, but how much time is reasonable to deal with the need for shelter, food, transportation and less obvious but vital requirements such as child care? Public service employees, including healthcare personnel, need clear and consistent guidelines if both their personal needs and those of the community are to be met with an appreciation for their pragmatic requirements.

Depending on the disaster's extent and duration, caregivers must receive periodic downtime to recover physically and emotionally to avoid burnout. Although replacement personnel may be available from other states, they will not be permitted to treat patients unless their credentials have been previously reviewed, they have been approved as members of the Department of Health and Human Services' Medical Reserve Corps, or until the governor requests and receives authorization from FEMA. There may be other legal and regulatory constraints that could impede the use of qualified volunteers, and the disaster plan should anticipate and address these constraints.

FACING COMMUNICATION CHALLENGES

Inaccurate and incomplete information severely compromises the ability of all parties to cope productively during a disaster. Given the enormous range and magnitude of communication issues associated with a catastrophic event, policies and procedures must consider the specific needs of individuals (patients, families, staff and volunteers) in addition to entities (communities, fire and police departments, government agencies and the media). We should not rely on the insight and intuition of a few key people regarding crucial linkages and practices; these matters must be well documented and the content easily accessible.

Most leaders are not eager to think about worst case scenarios and how to prepare for them, but they cannot relinquish their responsibility to ensure someone within the organization has done so. "Are Hospitals Disaster-Ready?" was the rhetorical question raised by the fall 2006 issue of ACHE's journal *Frontiers of Health Services Management.* The practical advice about emergency generators, evacuation issues, security needs, developing resilience and a host of other topics is essential reading. Leadership during disasters requires competence and resourcefulness, but effective leadership cannot occur unless it is preceded by creative and effective planning.

January/February 2008

The Ethics of Hospital Marketing

William A. Nelson, PhD, and Justin Campfield

Our facility is developing a marketing campaign in a competitive environment. Are there ethical guidelines for marketing?

In the increasingly competitive world of healthcare delivery, more and more hospitals are engaging in marketing to expand awareness of services that can build market share, diversify the payer mix, and generate needed revenues. But does the altruistic nature of hospitals make it inappropriate for them to market their services in the same ways companies in other sectors market their goods? Because of the perception that marketing is more about financial enhancement than enhancing a community's healthcare needs, is the term "marketing ethics" an oxymoron?

We, like others, take the position that marketing by healthcare facilities can be appropriate and ethical. Marketing can function as an extension of the organization's transparency by communicating its various services.

However, there are specific situations when marketing efforts either raise ethical questions or are, arguably, inappropriate, such as when the marketing message is less than truthful, is manipulative, or creates a conflict of interest. One example is the classic case of the hospital that was advertising it would provide free meals to ambulance drivers when they brought patients to their emergency room.

The basic ethical standards of marketing as described by the American Marketing Association include honesty, fairness, and avoiding conflicts that promote the organization's interest over consumer needs. These fundamental marketing ethical guidelines also are reflected in ACHE's *Code of Ethics*, which states: "Be truthful in all forms of professional and organizational communication, and avoid disseminating information that is false, misleading or deceptive."

In addition, the American College of Physicians *Ethics Manual* indicates that "advertising by physicians or healthcare institutions is unethical when it contains statements that are unsubstantiated, false, deceptive or misleading, including statements that mislead by omitting necessary information."

Adhering to ethical standards cannot be undervalued because of the inherent relationship between ethical practices and organizational success. Unethical marketing, whether real or perceived, can ultimately be harmful to the organization. So the issue is not whether it is ethical to market, but, rather, how does a healthcare facility do so ethically?

There is no simple, absolute answer to this question. However, the leadership of the healthcare facility, the group developing the marketing activity, and perhaps representatives from the healthcare facility's ethics committee should reflect on the following questions before any campaign is implemented:

- **Why is the marketing campaign being developed and potentially implemented?** Are the hoped-for results truly aligned with the mission and best interests of the hospital and the community it serves?
- **How does the service or activity being promoted address a community health need?** Is the marketing effort promoting the use of effective care—treatment viewed as medically necessary based on clinical-outcome evidence—rather than promoting

care because of the supply of resources or financial return? Is too much emphasis being placed on specialized care that can significantly enhance the facility's revenue stream compared to primary care services?

- **Is the campaign fully truthful? Is it misleading?** Unsubstantiated claims or needlessly concerning people about their health needs are not appropriate ways to promote a hospital.

- **Is the marketing activity fiscally responsible?** In a time of limited resources, is the marketing effort well matched to the community environment and an effective use of funds? For example, how will the spending of resources on four-color brochures and television advertisements be perceived versus supporting programs that meet the needs of the underserved? The marketing campaign should not take place in a vacuum, so if the talk of the town has recently been about a reduction in healthcare services, an increase in taxes (in hospital taxing districts) or a freeze in employee salaries, a marketing campaign may be seen by many as an unnecessary extravagance.

- **Does the tone of the marketing campaign fit the health-care organization's image and standing in the community?** As a provider of needed, life-saving services, hospitals should not market their services in the same ways as new cars or consumer goods. A question to consider is, will the marketing effort damage the facility's image in the community? The marketing effort should positively reflect on the healthcare facility's mission and culture.

- **If consumers know of the hospital only what they learn from the marketing campaign, are you OK with that?** There will be a segment of the local population that doesn't know much about you. A marketing campaign's ads and brochures may be all some consumers have as a basis on which to form an opinion of you. Do these materials send the right message?

In the end, the test is whether the marketing campaign will benefit the hospital/community. This is the final and most important question that should be addressed. If the campaign is being undertaken to educate the public about needed healthcare services or support a crucial program of the hospital, you are most likely ready to go forward.

Healthcare marketing is ethical when the general ethical standards of practice are maintained. The responses to the above questions are not an algorithm for determining ethical marketing practices; however, the questions do provide guidance for determining whether your organization's marketing effort has crossed the line of unethical behavior. As healthcare organizations have become more focused on organizational and business ethics, it is reasonable and important to think about the proper standards for your marketing efforts.

November/December 2008

The Myth of Promise Keeping

Paul B. Hofmann, DrPH, FACHE

All healthcare organizations have promises and commitments that are implicit in their relationships with their patients and families and the communities they serve. What are an executive's responsibilities for ensuring these commitments are kept?

When people make promises or commitments, they create predictable expectations that the promises will be kept. Too often, they are not. These failures may be relatively minor or quite serious. But when the promise or commitment is implicit and when it is from a valued institution, the consequences are almost always damaging.

It is clearly unethical for a healthcare organization to make an implicit promise without a conscious intent to keep it. Hubris is generally not responsible for producing eloquent and admirable vision, mission, and value statements. Instead, these documents are almost always the result of well-intentioned trustees, executives and physician leaders working diligently at a board retreat to create or refine a set of statements that will capture the essence of the institution's raison d'être, incorporating language that is succinct, meaningful, challenging, and inspirational.

Annual reports describe the institution's impressive achievements; fundraising efforts explain why donations are so vital to maintaining and expanding crucial programs; and marketing campaigns are designed to attract potential patients, employees, and physicians. At a minimum in each case, direct or indirect references to the mission statement are made. We would be surprised if they were not.

TYPICAL IMPLICIT PROMISES

Providing exceptional patient care, demonstrating service excellence, improving community health status, ensuring effective stewardship of resources, treating patients and staff with dignity, respect, and honesty—these are only some of the predictable elements found in many mission statements.

Irrefutably, these and comparable phrases are intended to convey a clear message to multiple stakeholders: The organization has defined its mission and is committed to meeting the expectations it has created by doing so; therefore, every mission statement represents an implicit set of promises. Nothing in the language suggests these promises will be kept only when convenient or when we have adequate personnel.

All our public expressions essentially have declared that our care will be safe, effective, efficient, timely, and patient-centered. Some institutions also have indicated they would minimize barriers to access and reduce healthcare disparities. But having set forth these goals, there is an obligation to evaluate how the hospital is fulfilling its mission on both the macro and micro levels.

Information has always been available on the micro level, based on responses by patients, employees, and physicians to questionnaires and surveys. Increasingly, information on a macro level is available through Hospital Compare and similar hospital rating websites.

HAVING GOOD INTENTIONS IS INSUFFICIENT

Unexpected obstacles can certainly interfere with our good intentions and those of others. Uncontrollable events may make it impossible to meet once reasonable commitments. However, we should quickly determine when explanations for unmet promises are actually rationalizations and inadequate excuses, whether made by others or ourselves.

People feel vulnerable, frightened, dependent, and even intimidated when they are hospitalized. It is disturbing to hear an increasing number of individuals, including physicians and other healthcare professionals, advising their relatives and friends to spend as little time as possible without an advocate physically present in their hospital room to minimize the possibility of clinical errors and ensure commitments are met. This is a sad indictment of our belated and still too marginally effective efforts to create and maintain an environment that inspires a patient's confidence, not fear.

Frustration, disappointment and often anger are some of the most obvious reactions of those who are among the daily casualties of promise-breakers. In an article, published more than 20 years ago, about the importance of caring, I wrote: "How often does a staff member say to a patient, 'I'll be right back with some ice chips, I'll be right back with your pain medication or I'll be right back to help you with your bath'? We all know that delays can be unanticipated and frequently beyond our control as caregivers. Yet, we frequently leave a trail of broken promises and unfulfilled commitments, again not intentionally but because the words flow so easily and casually."

IMPROVING PROMISE KEEPING

Trust, like integrity, is an important but fragile commodity that, once compromised, is very difficult to restore. Regrettably, there is no simple ethical recipe to propose or follow to guarantee a prompt reduction in broken promises.

On the individual level, avoid the temptation, often because it is easy, convenient, or expected, to make or agree to commitments you cannot keep. On the institutional level, meet with patients and families who have been at the hospital and listen to what they have to say about the institution, the responsiveness of the staff, and their feelings about patient safety issues.

Use role playing in training and educational programs to dramatize the significant consequences for patients and families of being dependent on the power, authority, and resources of someone who lacks initiative or responsiveness.

Make teamwork more than a slogan in your hospital. Team members should communicate with each other and work together to achieve tangible goals whether the goal is ensuring every patient is visited each hour, hand-offs are smooth or patients and families have the information and opportunities they need to participate effectively in patient care decisions.

Be open and transparent with your community about where your hospital needs to improve and share your plans for accelerating your progress; consider ways to involve the community in your improvement efforts.

Highlight the link between the organization's mission and the expectation of patients, families, staff, and communities that everyone associated with the institution will honor its commitments.

An organization's failure to fulfill a promise is not just irritating or disappointing; such behavior can have immediate and long-lasting ramifications. Every executive should challenge senior leadership to examine carefully how implicit promises pervade the institution's messages to determine where promises are not being kept and to develop action steps to close the gaps.

September/October 2008

Conflicts of Interest

William A. Nelson, PhD

CONFLICTS OF INTEREST are an increasing concern across almost every sector, including business, government, politics, finance, education, and healthcare. Newspapers are filled with stories of the fallout stemming from institutions and people involved in conflict of interest situations. Healthcare certainly is not immune to these concerns.

According to a 2005 survey of physician executives published in *Physician Executive*, 90 percent of the respondents were very concerned or moderately concerned about unethical business practices. Sixty-six percent of the respondents further indicated they were concerned about nonphysician executives and board members' conflicts of interest. As a result, healthcare facilities need to develop approaches for recognizing, managing, and preventing conflicts of interest.

DEFINING CONFLICTS OF INTEREST

Managing conflicts of interest requires a clear understanding of what the concept entails. A suggested definition is: Conflicts of interest occur when self-interest affects an individual's professional obligations to one's patients, organization, and/or profession. A similar definition states: Conflicts of interest occur when a personal or private interest influences (or appears to influence) a professional's objective judgment and the exercise of that individual's recognized duty.

Even lacking a uniform definition, the various definitions reflect the basic components for a conflict of interest to occur:

- **Self-interest and/or personal interest:** The self-interest often is described as financial, but it also can include providing a special advantage to a friend, business associate, relative, vendor, or supplier.
- **Professional and/or organization duty:** Healthcare executives are expected to be competent and fulfill their responsibilities in a manner that reflects their profession's standards, including its code of ethics. Additionally, executives and other healthcare organization staff have an obligation to direct their activities and decisions to fulfill the mission and values of their organization.

The conflict of interest occurs when one's self-interest or personal interest interferes with or alters objective professional judgments or actions. Healthcare professionals are respected not only because of their recognized competence, but also because they carry a public expectation that they will act on behalf of and in the best interest of patients and the organization's mission. Therefore, conflicts of interest undermine the fundamental fiduciary obligation of a professional and a healthcare organization to provide quality patient care.

Because everyone has a certain level of self-interest, such as wanting to receive an appropriate salary for a position, it can be unclear in certain situations whether a person's self-interest has crossed the threshold and is in fact a conflict of interest. Some have suggested a form of trust assessment because at the heart of conflicts of interest is a betrayal of trust. Ask yourself this question: Would your patients, employer, professional colleagues, the board, and the public trust your judgment regarding a particular decision or action if they knew you had a personal interest in it?

Ethical concerns also are raised when an individual's conflict of interest can, and most likely will, negatively impact the organization's integrity and commitment to its mission and value statements. In a very real and practical way, any conflict of interest will also lessen the community's image of the involved individual(s) and the organization.

PREVENTING CONFLICTS OF INTEREST

Directed by executive leaders, organizations should develop and pursue approaches to manage and prevent the occurrence of these detrimental situations. Several basic strategies have been suggested for preventing conflicts in today's healthcare setting. The article "Practicing Preventive Ethics—The Keys to Avoiding Ethical Conflicts in Health Care" by L. McCullough, published in *Physician Executive* (March/April 2005, 31(2):18–21), suggests the following:

- Continually emphasize and foster the fiduciary commitment of professionalism throughout the organization's culture and practices.
- Mission statements and policies should reflect an explicit commitment to the fiduciary responsibility of professionals and the organization to promote quality of care.
- Develop, implement and enforce a conflict of interest policy. The policy should be appropriately detailed, beginning with a statement of purpose and definition of the concept. The policy should include examples of conflicts of interest; require that all business, supplier, and vendor relationships be self-reported, including any gift and/or payment; describe the review process for assessing potential conflicts of interest; describe a method for others (whistle-blowers) to report a potential conflict; provide provisions for the enforcement of violations; and indicate the resources for clarifying the policy when needed.

Two additional components to a policy relate to managing potential conflicts. First, the policy should designate an office or person to guide clinicians or healthcare executives prior to accepting a relationship or activity with a healthcare supplier. Second, because disclosure of potential conflicts is essential, the review process should clarify whether the disclosed situation creates a conflict of interest for the individual or the organization.

Clearly not all relationships between administrators or clinicians and associations, businesses, or vendors create a conflict of interest. In some situations such relationships are beneficial. However, to avoid public misperception, the organization, after reviewing such situations through the conflict-of-interest policy review process, should publicly disclose all appropriate relationships with vendors, suppliers, and other business relationships, including payments received. One major medical center is developing a public website that will list all its staff's consulting arrangements, including the payments received. Such a high level of transparency, similar to the sharing of quality and outcome reports and the costs of healthcare treatments, fosters trust in the organization.

When drafting or updating a conflict of interest policy as suggested above, the ACHE ethical policy statement "Considerations for Healthcare Executive-Supplier Interactions," available on **ache.org**, should be used as a model resource.

Conflicts of interest are a serious concern that undermines the integrity of professionals and an organization's fiduciary responsibility to its patients and the community. An aggressive program that recognizes, manages and seeks to prevent conflicts of interest is essential despite the many complications that surround the concept of conflicts of interest. As with other organizational policies, an effective program to manage conflicts of interest can be achieved only through leadership that demonstrates the importance of avoiding conflicts of interest and supports a comprehensive educational effort propagating the policy and rigorous adherence to its implementation.

March/April 2009

Ethical Uncertainty and Staff Stress

William A. Nelson, PhD

ETHICAL UNCERTAINTY AND conflicts are encountered regularly by both healthcare executives and clinicians. There is a growing understanding that organizational and clinical ethical conflicts have a significant detrimental impact on today's healthcare organizations in many ways, affecting an organization's culture, quality of care, and potential for success.

Examples of the potentially harmful impact ethical conflicts can make on an organization include:

- **Staff:** caregiver stress, deflated morale, job turnover
- **Patients:** poor patient satisfaction, fewer self-referrals
- **Organizational culture:** diminished quality of care and professionalism
- **Relationship with community:** weakened organizational image, public relations and philanthropic giving
- **Legal:** increased litigation and settlements
- **Regulations:** negatively influencing adherence to Joint Commission and other regulatory organization standards
- **Organization's bottom line:** operational costs, diverted staff time, staff turnover; legal costs, settlements and malpractice premiums; and public relations and marketing costs, repairing

public image and loss of self-referrals in competitive markets (Nelson, W. A., W. B. Weeks, and J. M. Campfield. 2008. "The Organizational Costs of Ethical Conflicts." *Journal of Healthcare Management* 53 (1): 41–52).

MORAL DISTRESS

Staff members' moral distress is a major dimension of ethical conflicts. It appears that nurses in particular are affected by the phenomenon when dealing with the uncertainty surrounding ethical challenges. Andrew Jameton, PhD, a professor in the College of Public Health at the University of Nebraska Medical Center, first described moral distress among nurses in a nursing ethics book more than 20 years ago, but the issue has since received limited attention and is rarely discussed. Moral distress has primarily been associated with clinicians, but healthcare executives, managers, and staff members also can experience such distress.

There are several factors contributing to moral distress. One factor is ethical uncertainty, a situation in which a staff member is uncertain about the ethically appropriate course of action to take. The healthcare professional may keep this uncertainty to himself and not share his stress because he thinks he is alone in his uncertainty.

There also are situations in which the healthcare professional does raise ethics questions but feels unsupported in acknowledging her uncertainty and is without an available resource to share and discuss the issue. In both examples, the staff members feel alone in their uncertainty. In such situations, healthcare professionals can feel discouraged, frustrated, and isolated as they wrestle internally with their moral distress.

A different form of moral distress occurs when a healthcare professional knows or believes he knows the ethically appropriate course of action to take but is unable to carry out the action because of an organizational obstacle. The obstacle could be a supervisor, physician, or executive authority; lack of staff time; or legal or organizational constraints.

An obvious example is the nurse providing aggressive care, as ordered by the physician or the patient's family, while believing such a level of care is inappropriate in the given situation. Despite his misgivings, the nurse continues to treat the patient, leading to frustration, anger, and moral distress. Over a period of time moral distress can influence the staff member's morale, confidence, sense of purpose, integrity, and respect for the organization.

The findings from an empirical study using a moral distress scale noted a significant relationship between moral distress and staff satisfaction. In addition, 17 percent of the nurse respondents had left a nursing position and 28 percent considered leaving because of moral distress. The authors also noted the following relationship: the higher the level of moral distress the greater the likelihood of leaving a position (Hamric, A. B., and L. J. Blackwell. 2007. "Nurse-Physician Perspectives on the Care of Dying Patients in Intensive Care Units: Collaboration, Moral Distress, and Ethical Climate." *Critical Care Medicine* 35 (2): 422–29).

These findings confirm the perceptions and experiences of many in the healthcare field—that moral distress is real and can have a negative impact on healthcare professionals, the quality of care, and, due to high job turnover rates, the organization's overall financial situation.

DECREASING MORAL DISTRESS

Many factors can contribute to moral distress in the vertical hierarchy in which most clinicians and administrators function. These factors include differences in personal and professional values, organizational pressures, the lack of an effective ethics program promoting ethical practices, and lack of an ethical culture throughout an organization. To manage and potentially decrease the presence of moral distress and its negative effect on staff, organizations should take the following steps.

First, recognize that staff stress, morale issues, and even job turnover occurring in the organization may actually be the result of moral distress and ethical conflicts. Staff members should be self-aware of the phenomena and seek assistance. Equally, staff members should recognize signs of moral distress in colleagues. Recognizing moral distress can lead to constructive approaches for managing it.

Second, ensure an environment exists in which ethical questions or uncertainty can be openly shared and discussed. Leaders must create a culture in which all staff feel comfortable and safe to raise their ethical concerns, free from any retribution.

Third, ensure the organization's ethics committee is readily available to all staff members and that all are aware of how to access the committee. Ethics committee members should be knowledgeable about and skilled at addressing a broad range of potential ethical challenges, including organizational, management, research and quality improvement issues, besides the traditional clinical issues.

In addition to a reactive approach to moral distress, ethics committees should implement a proactive approach. Committee members should reach out to the various units of the organization and lead discussions to explore the scope and causes of recurring ethical challenges that create moral distress for the staff. Such discussions could lead to development of ethics practice strategies to address and possibly decrease the stressful nature of ethical conflicts.

Lastly, organizations need to ensure employee health programs are readily available to staff. Employees should be able to use these programs to discuss—in a confidential setting—emotional issues arising in the work environment.

Moral distress is real and has a negative effect on healthcare organizations. Healthcare leaders need to acknowledge this reality and, in conjunction with their ethics program leadership, develop and implement specific strategies for addressing the issue.

July/August 2009

PART III:

CLINICAL ETHICS ISSUES

CHALLENGES RELATED TO clinical issues arise within the context of clinician–patient encounters, often regarding what should be the appropriate course of action. Ethical conflicts occur when there is uncertainty, a question, or a conflict regarding competing ethical principles, personal values, or professional and organizational ethical standards of practice. This section consists of an exploration of many familiar yet challenging clinical conflicts that are regularly encountered in today's healthcare organizations.

The Executive's Role as a Patient Advocate

Sue G. Brody

*Recently, the interdisciplinary team evaluating our patient care plan-
ning process asked that I no longer attend meetings. They cited patient
confidentiality concerns. What do you think is the healthcare executive's
proper role in clinical matters?*

The ethical responsibilities incumbent upon healthcare executives are arguably more complex than those for any other role in our
field. Our position carries with it the responsibility to be our organization's chief patient advocate. As part of this function, we have
an obligation to attend to the best interests of each individual served
by our organization. This duty is, of course, shared by physicians
and staff directly involved in providing clinical care. But unlike those
providing direct care, the healthcare executive's role includes
another ethical dimension. In this position, we must also consider
our ethical responsibilities to our patients collectively, as well as to
our organization as a business concern.

Ideally, these responsibilities—to provide the best medical care
for each patient, to guarantee that every patient's medical needs are
appropriately met, and to ensure the organization's viability as an
ongoing business concern—should complement one another.
Often, they do. But in a competitive universe of limited resources

and a shortage of clinical staff, conflicts do arise. When they do, healthcare executives are responsible for resolving them. To do so, they must have enough information to properly consider the dilemma, weigh conflicting ethical interests, and make a decision that resolves the issue in an appropriate manner.

Some typical examples might include:

- Should scarce capital be used to purchase a piece of equipment that treats a small number of patients with a very serious illness? Or should those funds be used to buy a device that treats a larger number of moderately ill patients, even though other (albeit less effective) treatments exist?
- Should a hospital spend money on a much-needed emergency department renovation that would more effectively address the community's medical needs or use those funds to improve its balance sheet, thereby lowering the hospital's cost of debt and ensuring the financial viability of the organization in an era of stagnant revenues and increasing costs?
- Should the hospital fund a community outreach program that may identify those 'at risk' for a disease primarily treatable by a competing facility?

These decisions are important and cannot be made in a vacuum. How can healthcare executives properly perform their role as chief patient advocate if they lack specific information about the patient care process? How can executives properly weigh the interests of each patient, the organization itself, and their own responsibility to provide appropriate care to a patient population without an understanding of those interests? The answer is simple: They can't.

To properly discharge our ethical responsibilities, we have more than a right—as healthcare executives—to participate in patient care conferences and patient rounds. We have a responsibility to do so. Following are some strategies you may find helpful as you participate in patient care.

- **Define your role as chief patient advocate.** It is critical that physicians and clinical staff understand your role as chief patient advocate and its attendant ethical responsibilities, which include managing limited resources to provide the best possible medical care for each patient and ensuring the facility's ongoing financial viability. Make sure they have a proper context within which to view your participation in the clinical process. For example, your management and policy decisions will be made with a more profound understanding of the needs and priorities of those directly involved in clinical care because of your direct participation.

- **Identify opportunities to participate in the clinical process.** Find ways to become engaged in the clinical process that yield the greatest benefit for you—that is, ways that will help you make the most informed decisions regarding patient care. Ideally, these opportunities will provide an accurate representation of all your organization's clinical care processes. Some opportunities you may wish to consider are accompanying physicians on patient rounds, attending patient care conferences, participating in nursing unit staff meetings, and simply dropping by patient rooms to discuss their course of care with them.

- **Exercise your ethical responsibilities in a clear, unambiguous manner.** Make sure your administrative staff, as well as physicians and clinicians, understand how your ethical responsibilities affect your decision-making process. Make it very clear that ethical concerns, not simply financial ones, are important to you when making policy and executive decisions. This is an effective tool in demonstrating to physicians and clinical staff the practical value of your participation in clinical matters.

Preserving our patients' dignity and privacy is a matter of paramount concern. The new HIPAA regulations governing the disclosure of patient information run more than 1,500 pages. At the risk of severe oversimplification, I believe the new regulations can be summed up in one simple phrase: "Confidential patient information should only be disclosed to those with a demonstrated 'need to know.'" But healthcare executives clearly 'need to know' in order to properly discharge our ethical responsibilities and make the complex decisions that arise every day in the performance of our job. It is our responsibility to define and perform our function as chief patient advocate. No one else can do that for us.

May/June 2002

Making Life-Ending Decisions

Sister Irene Kraus, FACHE

RECENTLY MY ORGANIZATION expended considerable resources to treat a 30-year-old woman whose condition was deemed futile. Despite the care we provided and the resources we expended, she died within 12 hours of admission. In such situations, when resources are scarce, how can we determine when enough has been done?

The dilemma of the question being posed is: Are we prolonging life beyond what was and is considered morally and humanly acceptable?

For decades no one wanted to talk about death and dying. It was looked on as a fact of life no one wanted to face. Then came the boom in medical technology, which has allowed medical caregivers to actualize events that were once only dreams. Perhaps our technological progress has backfired on us.

From the ashes have risen new terms and new concepts, such as the "right to die." Is there truly such a thing? We have no choice whether we want to die. It's inevitable that we will. Of all the creatures on the face of the earth, only the human species is aware that it is dying. As a result, it would seem that we must make this event in our lives as sacred as possible. Nevertheless, that does not mean that we must use everything that is known to the medical profession to prolong life.

Families and caregivers must have norms to guide life-ending decisions. A balance must be struck between use of extraordinary means and costly procedures and the dignity of the patient, and the latter cannot be compromised. The decision to withhold or discontinue extraordinary or disproportionate means of medical intervention must be made with the judgment that the treatment itself is excessively burdensome or that the treatment is useless. It should never be made on the basis that the person's life is not worth living.

One ethicist, Elena Muller-Garcia, recently offered this advice: "Answering the following questions will help to determine when a treatment may be withheld or withdrawn:

- Is it too painful?
- Is it too physically damaging?
- Is it psychologically repugnant to the patient?
- Does it suppress too greatly the patient's mental capacity?
- Is the expense prohibitive?

If the answer to all of these questions is 'yes,' the extraordinary treatment may be withdrawn."

Sometimes families or caregivers are concerned that a course of treatment may be "useless" or "burdensome." This issue can only be addressed on an individual basis since what is useless to one person might not be useless to another. For example, what might be considered appropriate treatment for a 30-year-old who is terminally ill might be completely inappropriate for an 80-year-old. Aside from age, other possible norms might be whether the treatment brings about the effect for which it was designed (if not, it is medically inappropriate), the condition of the patient, and the benefit to be derived from the treatment.

Finally, patient concerns must be addressed regarding the decision whether to withhold life-sustaining treatment. I encourage everyone to have a living will, to have in writing what his or her desires might be relative to the established norms, to have a health "guardian" in the event that one cannot decide for oneself, and to have a dialogue with one's family, clergyman, and physicians before a life-and-death crisis occurs.

March/April 1996

Dealing with Noncompliant Patients

Paul B. Hofmann, DrPH, FACHE

We have a dialysis patient, with a history of mental illness, who peri-odically insists that treatment be discontinued. Often, this patient becomes verbally abusive and disruptive if treatment is not stopped. Is it ethically justified to force a patient to accept treatment?

Regardless of their mental status, patients will often decline treatment or insist that it be discontinued. As people become bet-ter educated about issues related to their care and more assertive in expressing their preferences, healthcare facilities should recognize that refusal to accept recommended therapy might become more common. To address these situations, healthcare organizations should develop noncompliant patient policies.

REASONS FOR DEVELOPING A POLICY ON NONCOMPLIANT PATIENTS

Each case will present its own unique set of circumstances, but handling every incident on an ad hoc basis will serve neither the patient's nor your organization's best interests. For at least three reasons, you should develop a policy on noncompliant patients before you need to apply it.

1. It is always preferable to create a policy in a noncrisis mode since myriad issues must be considered in dealing with noncompliant patients. The document should be prepared, reviewed, and refined in a time frame not compressed by the urgency associated with a specific situation.
2. A carefully constructed policy will always include input from your organization's attorney. Compelling a patient to accept treatment or alternatively, withholding or discontinuing treatment, could have obvious legal consequences. Certainly, you want to fully explore these issues before an evening or weekend telephone call to your on-call administrator.
3. A comprehensive policy provides direction and support to your staff and increases the likelihood that patients and their families are treated consistently. Healthcare professionals—including physicians, nurses, and social workers—are often morally stressed by noncompliant patients. As noted below, an effective policy will recognize that not only do patients have rights, but so does your staff.

ELEMENTS OF A NONCOMPLIANT PATIENT POLICY

Although the actual content of an organization's policy will vary—reflecting individual missions, values, and cultures—each policy should have common elements:

Preface

This general introduction should describe your policy's purpose. For example, it should acknowledge that patients and their surrogate decision makers may not comply with diagnostic or treatment plans;

in such instances, steps should be taken to preserve their rights and responsibilities, as well as those of staff. The comfort and safety of other patients must also be protected.

Definition of Noncompliance

A patient may be verbally abusive or physically combative or exhibit other behavior that makes it difficult and perhaps impossible to perform diagnostic or therapeutic procedures. Clarifying how patients are deemed "noncompliant" will help determine appropriate responses. Responses should vary depending on whether the conduct will irreversibly compromise the patient's clinical condition. The relative risks and benefits of intervention and nonintervention must be weighed. A distinction should be made between patients who exercise the right of autonomy via relatively "benign" noncompliance (refusal to eat a meal) and patients whose behavior significantly compromises others or whose level of nonadherence to a medical plan makes that plan futile.

Determination of Decision-Making Capacity

A patient could be legally incompetent to make an informed decision about his or her care—perhaps because of age, in the case of a minor, or as the result of medication, trauma, or disease. In the latter circumstances, patients can move in and out of decision-making capacity, so caution must be exercised to preserve their right to make an informed consent or refusal when justified. Options for assessing mental competency should be described.

Assurance of Continuity of Care

Regardless of a patient's aberrant behavior, your organization has a responsibility to maintain continuity of care. For example, you may need to arrange the patient's transfer to another unit within your organization or to a more suitable organization elsewhere. The policy should stipulate who has the primary role to explore and coordinate these arrangements.

Promotion of Patient Rights and Responsibilities

In addition to having the right to make an informed consent or refusal and to receive continuity of care, patients have other rights as well as responsibilities. These should be covered in a separate document on this topic, and it can simply be referenced in the policy or provided as an addendum.

Recognition of Staff Rights and Responsibilities

When employees believe their physical safety is being compromised, or verbal harassment has become intolerable, a procedure should be available so they can request prompt assistance with the immediate problem. This section of the policy should describe how a long-term solution will be provided if the relief is only temporary and the problem continues. It should also delineate your staff's responsibilities for addressing the needs of noncompliant patients.

Description of Available Resources

In addition to legal counsel, the potential role of your organization's risk manager, ethics committee, chaplaincy service, and other resources in dealing with a noncompliant patient should be explained.

Summary of Procedure

The policy should describe the sequence of activities necessary to achieve timely closure to the case. For example, first, be sure to document pertinent issues and discussions in the patient's medical record. Next, you may find it helpful to make a contract with noncompliant patients, describing expectations and related contingencies should inappropriate behavior continue. The responsible healthcare provider should also meet with the patient and, where appropriate, the patient's family (or others with a significant role in the patient's life) to discuss the consequences of continued noncompliant behavior before discontinuing care to an abusive, threatening, or uncooperative patient. Furthermore, you may want to delineate the use and content of a preliminary letter of warning and, if necessary, the use and content of a dismissal letter in your policy. Finally, there must be acknowledgment of the requirement, under federal law, to provide emergency care.

A RESPONSE TO THE DIALYSIS CASE

Forcing a patient to accept treatment under specific circumstances is ethically justified. Such circumstances would include a patient who

- is diagnosed with a life-threatening clinical condition,
- is a minor or legally incompetent because of illness or trauma,
- does not have an advanced directive that contraindicates intervention, or
- has a legally empowered surrogate who authorizes treatment.

Before taking any action, you should thoroughly review existing facts and collect missing information to ensure a comprehensive assessment of the issues and alternative actions. The safety of other patients and staff must not be jeopardized. You must also proceed in a manner that will avoid charges of abandonment or discrimination if services are terminated. The availability of a comprehensive policy on noncompliant patients, reflecting your organization's mission, culture, and values, should help create an ethical and appropriate response to these situations.

November/December 2000

Ethical Imperatives of Medical Errors

E. Haavi Morreim, PhD

In addition to the highly publicized Institute of Medicine report about the prevalence of medical errors, a number of other studies have brought greater attention to this issue. Acknowledging that traditional risk management programs are important but not sufficient, how can my organization respond to the ethical and legal imperatives to be more successful in reducing medical errors?

An error, according to the Institute of Medicine, is either a mistake in execution (the correct action did not proceed as intended) or a problem of planning (the intended action itself was not correct). Errors are not to be confused with risks or side effects, whose incidence is known but whose occurrence is not avoidable. To address the issues surrounding errors, we must distinguish ethical from legal imperatives.

ETHICAL IMPERATIVES

There are two major ethical imperatives: Avoid errors wherever possible and, when they do occur, do right by the people who are harmed. For avoiding errors, excellent ideas are now emerging, such as bar code drug delivery systems, integrated computer information systems, and blame-free error reporting followed by root cause analysis. Organizations should seek real and continuing improvement, not just window dressing.

Doing the right thing when an error occurs requires a broad view because patients are not the only ones who may be harmed. Physicians and other providers may be emotionally devastated in a medical culture that emphasizes perfection, self-reproach, and go-it-alone responsibility. When the error stems from ordinary human failings like fatigue, physicians' guilt may be undeserved; nevertheless it can impede their effectiveness in caring for patients in the future, as well as their willingness to participate in error-reduction efforts. Organizations need to help all staff cope effectively with those responses.

Where an avoidable error has led to significant harm or death, doing right by patients and families is, of course, the primary focus. Patients and families need to be told what happened, kept abreast of the investigation, and informed about efforts to prevent recurrences. Healthcare organizations should also offer reasonable compensation that will place those who are injured as close as possible to the position they would have been in had the error not occurred.

Not only is this the fair thing to do, but providing such information and assistance can yield two further benefits. First, only if patients and families know about the error can they provide additional information to assist in a root cause analysis that, in turn, might help prevent similar errors. Second, every risk manager has heard patients and families insist that "this must never happen to anyone else." Participation in the organization's improvement process can help those who have suffered from error to find personal value and meaning in a tragic situation.

LEGAL IMPERATIVES

The ethical imperative to help restore patients and families as close as possible to their "pre-error" state has the ring of tort law because, in this area, good ethics is also good law. The essence of fault-based tort law is not to extract money from the richest person. Rather, it is to make sure that innocent people do not have to bear the costs when they are injured by another's carelessness. Conversely, if no one is specifically at fault, then shifting the blame for the misfortune on organizations or individuals simply because they have "deep pockets" is equally unfair.

That is the ideal, at any rate. Today's judicial realities, however, do not always match this ideal. Courts are sometimes quick to find "fault" in the actions of whichever party has the money to help an injured patient.

There is nothing inherently wrong with prudent self-interest, although it should take a backseat to important ethical mandates. Fortunately, in this area there may not be as much conflict as organizations assume. *Annals of Internal Medicine* recently reported that one hospital's experience with "extreme honesty" was economically as well as ethically superior. After a single year in which two judgments alone cost $1.5 million, a Kentucky VA hospital began investigating errors thoroughly, informing patients and families when errors had caused injury or death, helping them to find legal representation, and then negotiating a mutually agreeable arrangement for restitution, compensation, and/or corrective action. After seven years under this new policy, the hospital's payouts for settlements and malpractice claims totaled only $1.3 million.

A flurry of studies over the past decade suggests that people often sue for reasons having little to do with medical negligence or even adverse outcomes. Rather, suits are commonly filed because of anger and poor relationships. In one study, 48 percent of mothers of dead or injured infants felt that the physician had actually tried to mislead them, and 70 percent felt that the physician had not warned them adequately regarding the infant's long-term problems. And many patients sue when they conclude that filing a claim is the only way to find out what really happened.

In the end, error reduction, combined with appropriate disclosure and compensation, appears to offer abundant opportunities in which good ethics is also good healthcare and good business.

July/August 2000

Navigating Differences in Patient Values

Paul B. Hofmann, DrPH, FACHE

My organization has encountered situations where differences arise between a caregiver and a patient's or family's preferences. Sometimes these differences directly affect the decision to provide or withhold treatment. How can such conflicts be resolved?

The question raises a host of issues reflecting the complex dynamics that influence patient care decision making and the role that patients, family members, physicians, nurses, and other healthcare professionals play in those decisions. Following are a few issues at the heart of treatment decision-making conflicts:

- Caregivers can intentionally or unintentionally impose their values and beliefs on their patients. Because patients often feel compromised by their clinical condition, dependent on caregivers, and intimidated by the hospital's bewildering complexity, they may be reticent and acquiesce too readily to a physician's recommendation, even when such a recommendation is not consistent with their own preferences.
- Caregivers may assume that patients share their values and beliefs. With pressures to reduce lengths of stay, staff often

have less time to develop a complete appreciation of their patients' convictions.

- Various participants in the treatment decision-making process may clearly express disagreement rather than acquiesce.

CAUSES OF CONFLICT

The reasons for disagreement are not always obvious. Conflict may be based upon genuine differences in culture, values, or beliefs; however, disagreement can occur over a simple misunderstanding due to poor communication. Even when medical jargon is assiduously avoided, the patient and/or family may still have difficulty understanding the physician's explanations and guidance. Disagreement can also be caused by the patient's anxiety, fear, or even anger related to the problems caused by the disease or trauma. Occasionally, the dispute could be related to a physician's reluctance to concede that continued aggressive diagnostic and therapeutic interventions would not prolong the patient's life expectancy or quality of life.

Other personal issues can complicate the decision-making process. The patient may be in denial about the prognosis, distrustful of the physician, convinced that a religious or medical miracle will occur, or involved in an interfamily quarrel. Perhaps surprisingly, a sense of guilt could be the basis for disagreement. For example, a family member feeling alienated by time or distance may insist that futile heroic measures be maintained or instituted because the relative feels guilty that he or she has not maintained a close relationship with the patient.

RELEVANCE OF ETHICAL PRINCIPLES

Autonomy—respecting the patient's right of self-determination—is a universally accepted ethical principle. If the patient lacks decision-making capacity, the patient's designated surrogate or proxy has the authority to act on the patient's behalf. It is assumed that this person would best represent the patient's personal preferences. Although caregivers may strongly disagree with the patient or the individual exercising "substituted judgment," courts have confirmed (with rare exception) the patient's prerogative to accept or refuse diagnostic or therapeutic procedures, and to decide who should be the proxy when the patient is not legally competent to make a decision.

Truth telling, fidelity, and promise keeping are three additional, closely related ethical principles that are relevant to these situations. If a caregiver anticipates that a patient or family's preferences are at variance with those of the caregiver, a different decision might be elicited by subterfuge, such as distorting information to ensure a more "appropriate" response. Similarly, a caregiver could assure a patient that his or her wishes would be followed not to institute resuscitation measures or, alternatively, to do everything possible, and then rationalize that contradictory actions were the result of misunderstanding by staff on another shift. Such behavior cannot be ethically justified in either case. Another critical ethical principle is nonmaleficence. Here the imperative is to do no harm. For instance, a physician or nurse may strongly object to a patient's decision and therefore refuse to administer or withdraw treatment. Under most circumstances, the caregiver has this prerogative, but not the option to abandon the patient. Instead, the healthcare professional has an ethical obligation to facilitate a transfer to someone who would be willing to continue caring for the patient.

ACCEPTABLE STRATEGIES

Resolving significant differences between a patient, family members, and/or caregivers is rarely easy or simple. A number of personal attributes will almost always be central to a successful resolution. Assuming there is consensus among the caregivers regarding the proper course, these attributes include

- insight about one's own values and acknowledgment that no one is value free,
- tolerance for values and beliefs that could be diametrically opposed to the caregiver's,
- sensitivity to the changing needs and expectations of participants trying to reach agreement on a course of action while struggling to cope with the consequences of disease or injury,
- patience to allow the patient and/or family members time to reflect on the advantages and disadvantages of pursuing a particular option, and
- persistence in working toward an acceptable conclusion.

Well-intentioned, compassionate caregivers, however, are not enough. Many conflicts are principally due to poor communication among the participants. People with special skills may be required to help clarify reasons for the disagreement, facilitate discussions, or mediate a perceived irreconcilable dispute. Colleagues, a chaplain, a language interpreter, a social worker, or an ethics committee member are among the organizational resources that may be useful.

It is important to recognize that patients and family members are not the only ones who feel stressed by conflicting opinions. Nurses, physicians, and other health professionals must have confidence that their organization appreciates the pressures under which they operate and through ethics grand rounds (i.e., educational programs focusing on specific cases), and other mechanisms, provides opportunities to explore creative techniques in a supportive environment.

March/April 2001

Promoting Complementary and Alternative Medicine Services

Elizabeth S. McGrady, PhD, FACHE

More and more payers and healthcare providers are responding to consumers by integrating complementary and alternative medicine into their services. Furthermore, I have noticed an increasing number of clinical studies showing the medicinal benefits of complementary and alternative medicine (CAM). What is my organization's— as well as my own—responsibility to develop, integrate, and promote CAM services?

During my research for a hospital consultation project, I asked an acupuncturist what she believed she could contribute to the provision of care in a hospital environment. While she offered several ideas, the one that caught my attention was her assertion that acupuncture significantly benefited stroke patients. She claimed that the sooner acupuncture is provided in such cases, the better. Thus, she believed that providing acupuncture in the emergency department setting is warranted.

As I found myself questioning her statement days later, I decided to examine references of clinical studies for acupuncture; I found five such studies documenting the benefits of acupuncture for stroke victims (Freeman and Lawlis 2001) and two that did not find additional benefits in addition to conventional rehabilitation (*Stroke* 1998, 2002). I also discovered that acupuncture has an even greater demonstrated benefit for the treatment of pain for conditions such as osteoarthritis.

Much like you, I began wondering why the use of this modality isn't more prevalent if it has such merit. And what is the role of the healthcare organization in promoting this treatment? I found it helpful to address these issues in the context of ACHE's *Code of Ethics*, the standards that govern our profession as healthcare executives.

THE HEALTHCARE EXECUTIVE'S RESPONSIBILITIES TO THE PROFESSION OF HEALTHCARE MANAGEMENT

In ACHE's *Code*, the standards listed under this statement alone present the conundrum facing healthcare executives in relation to CAM. For one, healthcare executives must comply with the laws governing their state, and the laws regarding CAM practitioners vary greatly. For example, as of this writing, only medical doctors are permitted to practice acupuncture in Louisiana. This section of the *Code* also suggests that we perform our duties with dignity and refrain from activities that could demean the credibility of the profession. One of the challenges of promoting CAM is that it is an all-inclusive term. It includes a diversity of practices that are based in science—though perhaps practiced primarily by another culture—and other practices that have not yet, and may never be, clinically tested. There may even be practices that are harmful or bogus. Thus, healthcare executives have an obligation to develop processes to research both the practice and the practitioner before CAM programs are instituted in their organizations.

THE HEALTHCARE EXECUTIVE'S RESPONSIBILITIES TO PATIENTS OR OTHERS SERVED, TO THE ORGANIZATION, AND TO EMPLOYEES

This section of the ACHE *Code* contains provisions that include a patient's right to self-determination. Currently, in most healthcare organizations, a patient does not have the option to receive acupuncture treatments—or any other CAM service—in an emergency department. Is that ethical? A key issue in offering these services is our responsibility to ensure safe care. We should advise patients not only of their rights but also of the possible risks. Unfortunately, as healthcare executives, we have not done a good job of educating ourselves about CAM services. Most medical schools are currently teaching CAM practices as part of the curriculum, but are healthcare administration programs and professional organizations doing the same? This lack of information denies our patients the right to determine if CAM services may be the treatment of choice for them. Because many hospitals are intimidated by the prospect of credentialing CAM practitioners, qualified, accredited, and experienced practitioners cannot be integrated into the hospital setting to provide such services.

CONFLICTS OF INTEREST

The most frequently expressed barrier to integrating CAM services into the hospital setting is the resistance of the medical staff. In my work as a consultant, I have been amazed at the resistance that some physicians have staged to their hospital's exploration of CAM. Some doctors have even threatened to move their practice to another setting if the hospital proceeded. Practically speaking, as things stand, there is not much benefit for individual physician practices to embrace CAM services. CAM services can sometimes compete with traditional allopathic medicine, and there does not yet appear to be a mass consumer exodus toward physicians who integrate CAM services. Thus, it may not be practical to look to the medical staff for leadership in the provision of CAM services. The conflict of interest for healthcare executives is that we may be denying CAM practitioners access to practice—and patients wanting these services—in an effort to appease our key admitters.

THE HEALTHCARE EXECUTIVE'S RESPONSIBILITIES TO COMMUNITY AND SOCIETY

Is our commitment as healthcare executives to provide leadership for certain kinds of healthcare services, or to do what is best for our community and society? Although as a nation we spend more per capita on healthcare than any nation in the world, the United States ranks 37th in terms of health status according to the World Health Organization. Are we truly being good stewards of our resources? If your organization's mission statement reads, "We will be the best-focused factory in the provision of tertiary, allopathic medicine," then the discussion is moot. But most vision, mission, and value statements include phrases such as "health promotion," "healing," "the whole community," "the whole person," and "mind, body, and spirit." We need to ask ourselves, "What did we say we were going to do, and did we do it?" This is not to say that healthcare organizations have a responsibility to subsidize CAM services beyond the usual working capital. Our guidelines in ACHE's *Code* state that we should ensure "reasonable access" to services. We should "participate in public dialogue, advocate solutions, and provide adequate and accurate information to enable consumers to make enlightened judgments and decisions."

No one would suggest that healthcare organizations blindly proceed with offering CAM services without performing due diligence on their safety and efficacy. Therein lies the problem. To proceed in a prudent manner, we will have to dig a little deeper and through new channels to learn what we need to know. Today, some CAM services are considered to be almost "mainstream" medicine; however, there are also CAM services that may have no merit or that are inconsistent—or even contraindicated—with their integration into traditional allopathic medicine. We probably won't receive much help from our medical staff in determining the difference, simply because they have not been trained, are resistant, or have no interest. Therefore, the ethical imperative is not only to be open to the idea of CAM. We must also become educated about which CAM services and providers are available and working in our area, and which services our customers want.

If I, or any loved one of mine, should have a stroke, I am willing to take my chances on a treatment that has no side effects, costs under $100, and may reduce the deleterious effects of this affliction; aren't you?

September/October 2002

Promoting Advance Directives

Paul B. Hofmann, DrPH, FACHE, and Bruce Jennings

The Terri Schiavo case dramatized the importance of having an advance directive that documents a person's preferences regarding life-sustaining treatment options. Federal law now requires healthcare organizations receiving Medicare and/or Medicaid funds to ask patients at the time of their admission if they have an advance directive and prohibits them from pressuring an individual into completing one. But, while still complying with the law, should these organizations be doing more to increase the proportion of all adults with such documents?

Regardless of one's personal views of the Schiavo case, one positive outcome was the tremendous growth in public awareness about the value of discussing personal preferences concerning end-of-life treatment options and designating a surrogate decision maker. An opportunity now exists, but this interest will dwindle over time unless a more aggressive and assertive campaign is mounted to ensure that advance directives are actually executed, placed in the individual's medical record, and then honored by health professionals.

BACKGROUND

Historically many hospitals have been hesitant to be aggressive in promoting the completion of advance directives, including documents described as durable powers of attorney for healthcare and living wills. This passive role of hospitals was not necessarily due to their traditionally conservative views of new social movements or being risk averse to taking a high-profile position that might generate public criticism. Instead, they have been very sensitive to the language of the Patient Self-Determination Act, the 1991 federal legislation requiring organizations receiving federal funds to ask adult patients about the existence of an advance directive. Healthcare organizations may not discriminate against a person who does not complete an advance directive; for example, the completion of advance directive forms cannot be a condition of admission to a facility. In addition, employees are explicitly prohibited from serving as witnesses if these documents are completed within the organization.

These constraints were a prerequisite to Congressional passage of the act at the time because, in part, they reflected the ambivalence and ongoing controversy in America about forgoing life-sustaining medical technology and allowing natural death. To accommodate opponents of the legislation, ensuring the "neutral" role of institutional providers was a vital concession. In the absence of such neutrality, at least some legislators felt that hospitals, nursing homes, and home health agencies might be viewed as having a hidden agenda, one designed to force patients and their families to make hasty and perhaps unwise decisions to limit life-sustaining treatment options. Others were categorically opposed to any provision that would seem to favor the right to forgo artificial nutrition and hydration, a form of treatment that some regard as basic and ethically mandatory.

GREATER ROLE BY HEALTHCARE ORGANIZATIONS

Society has paid a price for not recognizing the value of advance directives. Since 1991, when less than one out of ten adult Americans had advance directives, there has been a gradual increase in the perceived benefit of these documents. Even so, the total percentage of Americans who have signed an advance directive remains very low. Moreover, some studies have determined the presence of an advance directive and even a do-not-resuscitate order in a medical record does not guarantee that patients' preferences will be followed. Patients and families need more positive incentives to make better use of them, and physicians and other healthcare professionals need to comply with them consistently.

The lay press and professional literature have made a compelling case for completing advance directives. On a daily basis throughout the country, patients, families, employees, and physicians are severely compromised by the lack of clear and convincing evidence of patient preferences regarding not only end-of-life decisions, but also other medical decisions when patients temporarily lack decision-making capacity.

A patient's values and preferences, when not documented, are open to wide interpretation if the patient is unable to participate in decisions affecting his or her treatment. The potential for disagreement and conflict among family members and staff is much higher under these circumstances. Among other problems, a lack of consensus around a decision either to halt or continue treatment may provoke allegations of insensitivity, generate feelings of guilt, create increased stress, and produce threats of litigation.

RECOMMENDED ACTIONS

How can healthcare organizations become more aggressive in encouraging more people to have advance directives? Within the first five days after the American Hospital Association launched its "Put It in Writing" website (www.putitinwriting.org), it received more than 11,830 individual visitors who stayed an average of more than eight minutes. The AHA reported the wallet card was downloaded more than 4,150 times, and the brochure more than 3,550 times. Hospitals were encouraged to include a link on their websites to the AHA's site (www.aha.org), which contains resources to help people put their wishes about end-of-life care into advance directives.

One step already taken by many health systems and hospitals is to sponsor community forums and to collaborate with other organizations that help educate citizens about advance directives. Waiting to introduce the concept of an advance directive to a patient who has never been exposed to its purpose until an elective hospitalization causes unintended anxiety. Thus, there is wide agreement that physicians should discuss advance directives with patients during routine annual visits. Nonetheless, because healthcare organizations have greater visibility, more resources, and a community education responsibility, their leaders should be insisting that this topic be highlighted in local forums, as well as in newsletters to staff, volunteers, and residents in their service areas.

Since cultural and language barriers can undoubtedly impede the completion of advance directives, special efforts must be undertaken to help patients and families understand both why they exist and to dispel any fears or misconceptions they may have about them. Failure to do so is a sign of disrespect. Ethnic disparities in the provision of healthcare services and their outcomes are irrefutable. Failure to assist with advance planning and advance directives puts patients at risk for futile, burdensome, expensive, and unwanted treatment or, alternatively, denying these same individuals treatment when it would be desirable.

Finally, executives should devote at least some of their political leverage to this subject. Whether urging amendments to the Patient Self-Determination Act or taking similar actions to influence legislation and regulations at the federal and state levels, healthcare leaders

have an unprecedented opportunity to sustain the public's awareness of these complex issues and to promote more informed con-
versations around end-of-life treatment decision making.

September/October 2005

Making Decisions About Neonatal Life Support

Charles L. Stewart, FACHE

My hospital's Ethics Committee met with our staff neonatologists to discuss discontinuing advanced life support for a two-month-old infant born with severe physical abnormalities. The parents of the baby agreed with the physicians and the committee's recommendation. However, the nurses involved in caring for the infant disagreed with the recommendation and refused to follow the wishes of the parents. How can I resolve this issue in a manner that respects everyone's views?

A few years ago I experienced a very similar situation to the one you describe. Dealing with withdrawal of life support, particularly when it involves an infant, can be one of the most emotionally challenging ethical dilemmas that a hospital leader can face. In our example, a meeting of the Ethics Committee was called at the request of the staff neonatologists. The neonatologists recommended discontinuance of advanced life support for an infant with severe physical abnormalities who had been a patient in the neonatal intensive care unit for several weeks. The parents of the infant attended the committee meeting and expressed their desire to follow the neonatologists' recommendation. After a discussion and an assessment of the facts, the committee approved the recommendation, and the neonatal intensive care unit nurses were informed of the parents' decision. The nurses who had been involved in the care of the infant since her birth questioned the parents' wishes and the committee's decision. The nurses communicated to their nurse manager that they refused to participate in caring for the infant during her death. My initial reaction was "How could they refuse to follow the parents' request?" As administrator, it was my responsibility to honor the wishes of the infant's parents while respecting the moral and ethical dilemma the nurses faced and to somehow bring about a resolution that respected everyone's views.

I called a second meeting of the Ethics Committee and invited the nurses who were involved with the baby's care in the NICU. Five of the nurses who had provided care for the infant attended the meeting. I explained that the purpose of the meeting was not to make a decision about the fate of the baby but to open lines of communication between all parties. The nurses expressed that they did not feel they had been completely informed of the seriousness of the baby's condition. They did not believe that the parents had shown proper concern for the infant, as evidenced by the small amount of time that they had spent with the baby in the NICU. It was their belief that if the parents had really cared about the infant, they would have requested the baby be transferred to the regional children's hospital for additional evaluation and treatment.

The neonatologists explained the seriousness of the infant's condition to the nurses. They explained that because of difficulty with the lungs and abnormalities of facial structures, the infant's ability to breathe was impaired, and all attempts to remove her from a ventilator had failed. EEG activity had been abnormal at birth, and a report by a pediatric neurologist consulting on the case indicated uncertainties of the infant's potential intelligence and that quality of life was very unpredictable. The neonatologists explained that, in their opinion, the baby was suffering. They had discussed the seriousness of the condition with the parents as well as the option of transfer to another facility. The mother did not want to put the baby through more test procedures or suffering when there was so little hope for improvement. The father's main concern was the quality of life for the infant.

The director of Social Work explained that she had counseled the parents during the baby's hospitalization. She had observed that the baby's condition had been very difficult for the parents. Initially, the parents had spent a great deal of time at the hospital, but as time went by the parents had visited less frequently. The social worker explained that, in her opinion, what had appeared to be a lack of concern on the part of the parents was actually their defense mechanism for avoiding hurt and further attachment to the infant. The parents were young and unmarried and held low-paying jobs. The social worker was initially concerned with the amount of time the parents were spending with the infant; however, she had come to believe they deeply cared for the baby but were emotionally torn between being with the infant and needing to maintain their income.

The attorney informed the committee that state law was clear that an adult has the right to make medical decisions for himself or herself, but it was not clear as to what parents or other responsible parties can or cannot do in a situation such as this. The attorney expressed that there was no legal reason not to follow the parents' wishes. The social worker explained that she had initially questioned the parents' ability to make a proper decision and that she had contacted the state's Department of Human Resources to assume state guardianship of the infant. The state department had refused to get involved.

It became abundantly obvious that our well-intentioned structure designed to address this type of issue had been seriously compromised by a lack of coordinated communication between all parties. Those who had been most intimately involved in the care of the patient—the nurses—were the least aware of most of the facts. I complimented the nurses for their compassion and commitment to their patient. I agreed with their suggestion that we should seek a second opinion and agreed that the hospital should bear the expense. I believed this was necessary to achieve consensus among the family, committee members, and nursing staff. A second opinion was obtained at the regional children's hospital, but it revealed no new information. The baby was transferred back to our hospital, where the nurses then accepted the condition.

As hospital leaders, we have a responsibility to our organization to learn from our mistakes. In our attempt to resolve the issue in a manner that respected everyone's view, we identified three areas that needed improvement:

1. **Communication.** When the nurses met with the committee, we learned that the neonatologists had not communicated the condition of the infant to the nurses, creating a false expectation among them. The social worker had come to understand the family dynamics but had not shared this information with the nurses. Team conferences were instituted to overcome the communication barriers between nurses, neonatologists, and social workers. The Ethics Committee composition was changed to include direct caregivers of the patient whenever necessary.

2. **Policies and procedures.** Policies and procedures are the guides that staff look to when problems arise. When faced with the dilemma, we realized that our policies and procedures fell short as to the rights of minors and parents. Even state law offered no clear direction. It also highlighted the need to review the rights and responsibilities of employees.

3. **Education.** The need for greater awareness of cultural differences was made evident by the nurses' perception of the parents' behavior. Their initial refusal to participate in allowing the baby to die was insensitive to the parents' feelings and wishes. To better prepare the nurses to deal with their emotions and personal differences, we utilized counselors to provide training in conflict management and diversity. Open dialogue about diversity can help staff be better prepared when faced with a real event.

March/April 2005

Accountability for Nosocomial Infections

Paul B. Hofmann, DrPH, FACHE

The development of a nosocomial (hospital-acquired) infection is a classic example of an iatrogenic incident in hospitals and nursing homes. Within my organization, I suspect some patients are not informed that the infection is unrelated to their admitting condition, unless they are already debilitated, and are unaware of the additional length of stay it causes. What are the ethical, legal, and financial issues that this topic raises, and how should they be addressed?

This complex problem has only recently begun receiving the attention it deserves. More than five years have passed since the Institute of Medicine reported that up to 98,000 patients die each year in hospitals due to clinical errors. Yet this large number did not include all of the estimated 88,000 deaths that occur as the result of nosocomial infections, which affect approximately two million patients annually. Because a third of these infections are the direct result of acts of commission and omission, they should be viewed as clinical errors as well.

Ironically, some perverse financial benefits often accrue to the organization when an infection happens. In more than 100 DRGs, a hospital-acquired urinary tract infection causes the patient's care to be classified as "complicated." Consequently, although hospital-acquired infections are mostly preventable, reimbursement to the hospital can almost double when they occur.

One of the most frequently omitted actions by caregivers is the simple act of hand washing. According to the CDC and the U.S. Department of Health and Human Services, strict adherence to hand-washing procedures alone could prevent the deaths of 20,000 patients each year. When the implementation of basic, inexpensive measures can have such an enormous impact, there is no excuse for not taking immediate action. We have the ability to prevent many infections from occurring and others from spreading, for example, methicillin-resistant *S. aureus* infections. Failing to do so is ethically indefensible. What inhibits hospitals and caregivers from ensuring that everyone is more vigilant?

ORGANIZATIONAL BARRIERS

Historically, a variety of organizational barriers, as well as human nature, have impeded more rapid progress in reducing nosocomial infections. These include:

- **Denial and rationalization.** It is relatively easy to avoid taking strong action when the problem either is not acknowledged or is viewed as one of the unavoidable risks of being hospitalized.
- **Failure to establish a culture of safety.** Unless organizations empower employees, physicians, and even patients and families to identify the risks of infections, important and indeed essential allies will have been ignored in dealing with this continuing challenge.
- **Culture of blame.** As opposed to a culture of safety where emphasis is placed on teamwork and preventing harm to patients, a culture of blame focuses on individuals and reprimands them for causing the harm. When this happens, out of fear of retribution, staff members are much less likely to

acknowledge a mistake and suggest what can be done to avoid a recurrence.

- **Fear of liability.** Reticence to identify deficiencies is a classic component of a culture of blame, and this reticence is reinforced when there is a fear of punitive action in the form of legal action against the organization or the individual.
- **Inadequate education and training.** While everyone should be aware of the benefits of hand washing, providing repeated reminders about its importance helps achieve compliance. In addition, staff involved in the care of high-risk patients (for example, those in intensive care units) need to be carefully trained in the handling of intravenous lines and the changing of dressings to prevent infections. (For a case study in reducing catheter-related bloodstream infections, see page 20 of the March/April 2005 issue of *Healthcare Executive*.)
- **Resistance to change.** It is human nature for people to adopt habits or ways of performing their jobs that are convenient for them. These individuals are often unenthusiastic about modifying their behavior, particularly if they view the changes as interrupting their normal pattern of activity.
- **Deficient physical plant design.** Hand washing should be easy to do, especially now with alcohol-based hand rubs. However, sinks, alcohol-based hand rubs, and hand-washing solutions are often not close to the site of patient care and not readily convenient for use by caregivers.
- **Resource constraints.** Outmoded facilities, substandard staffing, and budget limitations make it more difficult to isolate infected and immunosuppressed patients, permit staff to follow and monitor proper infection control techniques, and purchase required equipment and supplies.
- **Lack of leadership and accountability.** Ultimately, the largest organizational barrier—as is usually the case with addressing any critical program—is the failure of administrative and clinical leaders to insist that this issue must be a high priority.

RESOLVING THE DILEMMA

A number of studies have now confirmed the obvious: Patients and their families recognize that even very competent staff members are fallible and make mistakes, but patients and their families do not understand, nor will they tolerate, cover-ups. Fortunately, they can be very effective allies in the patient care process. For example, asking staff members (physicians, nurses, or others) if they have washed their hands before conducting examinations, changing dressings, administering medication, and drawing blood can and does produce a marked improvement in hand-washing compliance.

Effective January of this year, the Joint Commission on Accreditation of Healthcare Organizations instituted new standards to cause facilities to focus more intensively on infection control procedures. All hospitals now must demonstrate compliance with hand-washing practices established by the Centers for Disease Control and Prevention. Providers are also required to report as a sentinel event, and submit a plan of correction for, each identified case of unanticipated death or major, permanent loss of function associated with a nosocomial infection.

Acknowledging a mistake or problem has occurred, genuinely apologizing for it, describing precisely what measures have been taken to avoid or minimize recurrence if the probable cause is known, and—when suitable—offering some reasonable compensation are steps in a response that has two distinct advantages. First, it is the most ethically appropriate response, at least in part because this is the manner in which you or a member of your family would want to be treated in a similar situation. Second, unless legal counsel advises to the contrary, it is most likely to reduce the likelihood of a lawsuit and the financial costs associated with defending a potential malpractice case.

Any adverse event affecting a patient's treatment and/or length of stay is lamentable. Discussing the event in a timely and forthright manner with the patient is an ethical imperative that is also a legally and financially sound practice, and it should be included in every organization's policy on disclosing clinical mistakes.

Now and in the future, we must continually ask ourselves why patients must suffer not just from injury or disease but also from their treatment. Only by having everyone focusing on preventing harm from occurring to patients will the incidence and sad consequences of preventable nosocomial infections be eliminated.

May/June 2005

Responding to Clinical Mistakes

Paul B. Hofmann, DrPH, FACHE

Despite everyone's best efforts to prevent medical errors, some mistakes will still occur. Considerable attention has been devoted to the role of physicians in dealing with this issue, but what is management's role?

The public is increasingly aware of the potential problems patients may encounter during hospitalization and outpatient treatment. Based on the findings of the Press Ganey 2005 National Healthcare Satisfaction Report, the greatest concern of patients is not privacy, tests, treatments, or staff but the hospital's response to their concerns and complaints.

To maintain the public's trust in our healthcare institutions, the organization has an irrefutable obligation to promote patient safety by taking every practical step to prevent mistakes. But this is not enough. Management has an additional responsibility to establish a comprehensive policy that is consistently applied when errors happen.

PIVOTAL QUESTIONS FOR SETTING POLICY AND PROCEDURES

Prior to developing policy and procedures regarding clinical mistakes, a number of critical questions should be considered. These include:

- How should the organization's vision, mission, and core values influence the disclosure of errors and the actions taken?
- How will the policy ensure that a patient-centered approach is promoted in dealing with errors?
- What constitutes a clinical error that should be disclosed?
- Are errors that have no measurable impact on patients addressed differently from those that do?
- What will be the roles of the nursing staff, risk management office, compliance office, human resources department, legal counsel, administration and public affairs office?
- What is the role of medical staff members?
- What should be communicated to patients and families when an error occurs, and who should be speaking with them?
- Under what circumstances does the organization communicate with other staff members, the governing body, outside regulators and the media?
- What information will be released, to whom and when? How are such communications handled?
- How will the organization deal with the individual(s) involved in the error in a blame-free and just culture?
- How will the organization address the system deficiencies that account for most mistakes?
- Is it necessary to provide a safe and anonymous means for staff members to report errors that have not been reported previously?

And regardless of such steps, what is required to ensure retaliation will not be permitted or tolerated?

- What mechanisms have been developed to support proper involvement of patients and family, timely root cause analyses and other steps to reduce clinical mistakes?

A policy on disclosing clinical mistakes should begin with a preface that describes not only its purpose but also why the institution's core values mandate compliance with the policy. The preface should note the importance of (a) recognizing that errors will happen, (b) acknowledging them and apologizing when they do, (c) performing thorough investigations, and (d) taking steps to minimize future mistakes. The balance of the policy and the accompanying procedures should address the questions raised above.

THINK FIRST OF THE PATIENT AND FAMILY

One simple litmus test should be used in evaluating the policy's adequacy and relevancy: If you were the patient who had been hurt by a clinical error or were a member of that patient's family, what would be your expectations?

First, you would want acknowledgement that a mistake was made. Moreover, this disclosure should be prompt, accurate, and in terms you can understand. Specifically, you deserve to know what happened, how it happened, what are the consequences for you, whether those consequences are temporary or permanent, and who will be responsible for the incremental costs associated with any necessary treatment. As important, you would not want the disclosure to be delayed until every single detail of the error is known. This is a predictable tendency of healthcare organizations but not one that meets your need for timely disclosure and a promise of more information when it is available.

Second, you would expect an apology. And of course, it should be genuine and candid, not scripted and impersonal. Because you did not anticipate being harmed during your hospitalization or out-patient visit, you will be upset. If someone says they are sorry and expresses sincere regret, patients and families will still be angry, but their anger may be partially dissipated by an admission of remorse. People understand mistakes can happen; they do not and should not need to understand why no one has accepted responsibility, admitted there was a problem, and apologized for it.

Third, you would expect to be informed about steps underway to investigate why the error occurred and what measures will be taken to prevent similar errors from recurring. It may be small solace to know others will be at less risk in the future, but patients and their families can be somewhat comforted by this knowledge.

Fourth, you would expect a preliminary indication that some form of compensation will be forthcoming. Although still subject to debate, risk managers and healthcare attorneys are aware of growing evidence that both the likelihood of a lawsuit and the size of settlements often are diminished when a timely and appropriate offer is made to compensate for the pain and suffering associated with the mistake.

FINAL THOUGHTS

Healthcare institutions are belatedly encouraging and promoting the concepts of transparency and disclosure. Working diligently to acquire and retain the public's trust, hospitals and other providers should remember that patients and families realize staff members are fallible and some mistakes inevitably will occur. However, these same patients and families also share the view of Sir Liam Donaldson, chief medical officer of the United Kingdom Department of Health: "To err is human; to cover up is unforgivable; and to fail to learn is inexcusable."

September/October 2006

The Ethics of Patient Preferences

William A. Nelson, PhD

Patients often demand treatments, medications, or specific clinicians. Are there limits to patient determination?

During the past few decades, there has been an evolutionary shift toward the importance of patient autonomy within the clinician–patient relationship. Patient preferences are the foundation for informed consent based on a shared decision-making process.

Despite the importance of these preferences in decision making, however, patients do not have absolute authority. There are situations when it might be morally justifiable for a clinician to deprive the patient of his or her autonomy or situations when an organization's policies and procedures dictate the loss of patient autonomy.

Healthcare professionals are not obligated to carry out actions—such as providing treatments that are deemed unorthodox and lack a scientific basis—that contradict their basic goal to promote health by preventing or curing disease. In the informed consent process, the clinician's goal is to apply his or her medical knowledge and skills to promote the health of the patient.

A patient—or the patient's surrogate when the patient's decision-making capacity is lacking—can accept or refuse a recommended treatment presented in the consent process based on his or her personal preferences or values. In this situation, assuming the patient or surrogate is legally responsible for his or her decisions, the patient's preferences should determine whether the proposed treatment will be provided.

It is quite a different situation when the patient requests or demands a treatment outside the realm of those regarded reasonable by the clinician, such as an unorthodox treatment, unproven medication or unnecessary surgery. The clinician may consider the requested treatment but is not morally required to provide it if it is medically inappropriate or lacks a scientific basis for effectiveness, thus putting the patient at potential risk. The clinician's refusal to accept the patient's demand or preference in this case would reflect the overall goal of acting in the patient's best interest.

Another situation in which clinicians are justified in limiting patients' preferences is when a patient requests an unlawful action. For example, a patient may request that the physician not report a state-mandated medical disorder to the Department of Motor Vehicles. Or, a patient may request that the clinician certify a disability—even though the patient lacks such a disability—thereby allowing the patient to obtain a handicapped designated parking permit.

Despite the importance of patient preferences in healthcare decision making, these preferences do not impose an absolute obligation on the part of healthcare clinicians to act in a manner that is contrary to health professionals' medical or legal judgment.

More problematic are situations in which patient preferences challenge the clinician's personal values or the organization's values. These requests can range from a patient indicating that he or she only wants to be examined by a male or female physician to a patient refusing care from a provider because of race or sexual or religious orientation.

Although it rarely would be appropriate to accommodate such requests, a careful review of the circumstances can result in exceptions. When there is a medical basis for the patient's preference and a clear medical need, healthcare facilities should try to make a reasonable effort to accommodate patient preferences.

For example, a female patient demands that care be provided by a female rather than a male physician because the patient has been sexually abused by a man. After realizing the reasons behind the patient's request, the clinician should attempt an accommodation when an appropriately qualified female physician is available. If no qualified female physicians are available and there is no acceptable alternative to the patient's request (such as the presence of a female nurse), the patient should be informed of the situation with regard to his or her need for medical care. At this time, the patient also should be made aware of all available alternative options, including receiving care at another time or facility when or where the patient's preference can be accommodated.

The situation is more difficult when the patient's desire for a specific clinician is based on cultural or racial prejudice. In such cases, the clinician should attempt to reason with the patient, exploring the basis for the preference and reassuring the patient that the clinician is medically competent in addressing the healthcare problem.

While the hospital should not be put in the position of appearing to endorse the patient's prejudicial personal views, if a discussion with the patient is not successful, a reasonable effort should still be made by the hospital and clinician to provide the patient with needed care. As Jonsen, Siegler and Winslade pointed out in their book *Clinical Ethics*, healthcare ethics require that clinicians withhold or at least limit their moral judgments about patients regarding medical care. A clinician provides care for the wounded assailant as well as the injured assaulted person.

If, however, the patient refuses to receive care from the clinician, then the risks of not accepting the needed care should be thoroughly reviewed with the patient.

Despite employing this line of reasoning, there may be rare occasions when the healthcare professional's own personal values would not allow him or her to participate in patient care that is medically and legally acceptable. For example, a nurse may choose not to participate in an abortion or a terminal patient's desire to have artificial feeding and hydration discontinued. Organizations should have policies and procedures to guide and review a clinician's conscience-based desire to not participate in a patient's care.

The ethical conflicts surrounding the role of patient preferences in decision making can be challenging. Patient preferences and values are central to all treatment decisions; however, they do have limitations, such as when they are contrary to medical judgment, illegal, or contrary to a clinician's ethics. When patient preferences create ethical conflicts, the clinician should balance his or her aversion for the patient's values with the patient's need for healthcare.

As with other recurring ethical issues, the healthcare facility should proactively develop guidelines for addressing these conflicts and have a competent, readily available ethics consultation service to clarify those guidelines when individual cases arise.

September/October 2007

Ethical Questions at
the End of Life

Paul B. Hofmann, DrPH, FACHE

*Although polls consistently indicate people would prefer to die at home,
80 percent die in hospitals, nursing homes, and other facilities. What
are some of the key ethical questions related to healthcare at the end of
life, how should they be addressed and why should executives be concerned about them?*

Many elderly people are frightened about the possibility of
dying in pain, away from loved ones and hooked up to machines.
Their fear may be justified because more than 20 percent of terminally ill patients die in ICUs, although nine of ten people say
they would prefer a "low-tech" approach to their treatment at the
end of their life. Most people subscribe to Woody Allen's view, "I'm
not afraid of dying—I just don't want to be there when it happens,"
but this uncomfortable topic requires increased attention. For
example, advance directives are being promoted to encourage
adults to record their preferences regarding treatment options and
to designate decision makers when they lack decision-making
capacity ("Promoting Advance Directives," *Healthcare Executive*,
September/October 2005, pages 28–30), but the proportion of
Americans who have completed such documents is still less than
one out of five.

As healthcare professionals, we must be concerned first with meeting the needs of patients and their families. And yet, if we ignore the needs of employees and physicians who care for the critically ill and dying, they will be less effective in their roles as caregivers. At least one hospital documented that its highest nursing turnover occurred in the units that had the highest mortality, a situation it was able to correct by providing training in pain management to all nurses and offering a palliative care consultation service. Executives should champion both existing and new services that better serve critically and terminally ill patients and their families.

Literally hundreds of ethical questions can be raised concerning end-of-life care. Those that follow are purposely provocative and intended to stimulate a continuing dialogue among executives and clinicians about issues that demand continuing reflection.

REPRESENTATIVE END-OF-LIFE ETHICAL QUESTIONS

- Why is dying in America so hard? When the mere availability of technology makes its application our default position without adequate patient and/or family consultation, when pain and symptom management of terminally ill patients is inconsistent, and when studies have documented the frequency with which do-not-resuscitate orders are disregarded, the need for improved education, communication, coordination, and quality assurance programs is indisputable.
- How has families' concern about hospital treatment of terminally ill patients shifted? For years, in disputes over how aggressively to treat critically ill patients, families pressed to let their loved ones die, while physicians tried to keep them alive. More recently, the most common cases coming before hospital ethics committees involve families insisting on treatment that doctors believe is unwarranted.

- Why is a good clinical outcome not always desirable or appropriate? Usually, good clinical and patient outcomes are completely aligned, but success in prolonging organ function is not necessarily compatible with success in supporting a good death.
- Where is the best place to die? Although the vast majority of Americans die in institutions, most would prefer to die at home. Nonetheless, dying at home is not always practical, and ultimately a hospital death may feel safer, more comfortable, and more appropriate from the perspective of both the patient and the family.
- What is a good death? Dr. Richard Smith, former editor of the *British Medical Journal*, has written, "What is clear about a good death is that one size won't fit all. We want to be as different in dying as in living. Some want it sudden, some slow. Some want a quiet death with minimal medical involvement. Others want to follow Dylan Thomas and 'rage, rage against the dying of the light,' squeezing every last drop from life."
- What factors are considered most important at the end of life by patients, family, physicians, and other caregivers? All four groups rate five items the highest: pain and symptom management, preparation for death, achieving a sense of completion, decisions about treatment preferences, and being treated as a 'whole person.'
- What are the key ethical issues related to the administration of fluids, nutrition, and pain management for dying patients? According to the law, hydration and tube feeding are comparable to other treatments, and competent adults have the right to refuse treatment, as do their surrogates. Legally and ethically, there is no distinction between withholding and withdrawing treatment, but there is a difference psychologically and emotionally. Consequently, we must be sensitive to not only the concerns of the patient but also those of family members and staff. Pain management and heavy sedation are acceptable even if they hasten death

as long as the primary objective is to reduce suffering and not cause death.

- How can we be more effective in addressing value conflicts involving patients, families and staff? Predictably, more and better education is essential. Staff must realize that cultural humility and sensitivity are prerequisites to cultural competency; this includes understanding the attitudes and customs about death, medical care, and family interactions in the populations being treated. To a large degree, improved communication with patients and families depends on enhancing our listening skills. Too many health professionals think communication occurs when they are talking.

ADDITIONAL OBSERVATIONS

Some healthcare executives are not comfortable dealing with topics related to end-of-life issues unless they have a clinical background. Being a clinician such as a physician or nurse, however, is not necessary to be actively engaged in promoting effective end-of-life care. What is necessary is recognizing the validity of medical ethicist Howard Brody's observation, "Medical ethics is about power and its responsible use."

Dr. Brody's comment reminds us that the patient care playing field is very uneven, and executives as well as clinicians need to work hard to balance it. This is especially true when at least half of all patients do not make decisions for themselves as the end of their life approaches. Better staff training and more programs to ensure that the values of patients and their families are honored and respected are steps in the right direction.

January/February 2007

Ethics and Quality Improvement

William A. Nelson, PhD, and Paul B. Gardent, CPA

Is there a relationship between quality improvement activities and ethics in today's healthcare organizations?

The focus on the quality of healthcare has grown dramatically throughout the past decade. Though respondents to ACHE's annual Top Issues Confronting Hospitals survey continue to identify financial issues as the uppermost issue for CEOs, concerns related to quality and patient safety continue to gain prominence. In 2007, quality was noted as a top concern by 33 percent of respondents, increasing from 23 percent in 2005. Similarly, patient safety's placement as a top issue among the healthcare executives surveyed rose to 29 percent in 2007 from 20 percent in 2005.

Quality and safety of care is an expectation of all patients and is typically a prominent part of a healthcare facility's mission statement. Patients also expect that the delivery of their care will be ethical, and this is often described in a healthcare organization's value statement and code of ethics. We suggest that the expectation for and the goal of delivering ethical and quality care reflect a strong and interdependent linkage between the two concepts. Quality care is built on ethical standards and principles, and ethical practices foster quality care—the two cannot be separated. Just as quality and ethics are linked, so should healthcare programs and quality improvement efforts. This interdependent relationship between ethics and quality can be seen in several ways.

ETHICS IS THE FOUNDATION OF QUALITY

Several fundamental ethical principles drive the goal of providing high-quality healthcare. The principles are: autonomy (do not deprive freedom), beneficence (act to benefit the patient, avoiding clinician or executive self-interest), nonmaleficence (do not harm), justice (fairness and equitable care), and do your duty (adhering to one's professional and organizational responsibility). These ethical principles are the foundation for a healthcare organization's mission, staff members' values and clinicians' professional activities.

Adhering to these principles and organizational values is required to ensure quality care and patient safety. It is an organization's mandate, just as it is clinicians' and executives' professional responsibility, to ensure that quality care is achieved in all patient encounters. Therefore, ethics is the driver behind the goal of quality healthcare.

ETHICS IS THE FOUNDATION FOR THE DEFINING DIMENSIONS OF QUALITY CARE

The Institute of Medicine's report, *Crossing the Quality Chasm: A New Health System for the 21st Century*, describes the key dimensions of care that need improvement. Care should be: safe, effective, patient-centered, timely, efficient and equitable. These requisites of quality care are not only synergistic with ethics, but ethical concepts and reasoning are the foundation behind most current definitions of healthcare quality. For example, a patient-centered approach to healthcare means providing a respectful adherence to the patient's preferences and values through a shared decision-making process.

Such an approach is based on the ethical principles of autonomy and self-determination and is delineated in most healthcare organizations' ethical standards of practice, an informed consent policy.

Equity, another aspect of quality care, reflects an ethical understanding that all patients should receive quality care regardless of their personal characteristics such as gender, geographic location (e.g., a large, urban facility versus a small, rural facility), or socioeconomic status. Equity is based on the ethics concepts of distributive justice and fairness.

QUALITY IMPROVEMENT EFFORTS SHOULD REFLECT ETHICAL STANDARDS

During the past decade there has been significant focus on strategies to improve quality and safety of patient care and help the facility attain the key dimensions of quality. Just as clinical care and research should meet ethical standards, so should quality improvement efforts. Ethical concerns can arise when quality improvement activities cause harm or use resources inappropriately.

When a quality improvement effort is considered research, the activity will need to be reviewed according to federal regulations to ensure ethical standards are addressed. Participating patients will likely need to consent to such a research quality improvement effort. Even in situations where the quality improvement effort does not involve human subjects' research, such as a data-gathering activity, the activity should be undertaken in accordance with ethical standards.

Some of the specific ethical standards that have been proposed for all quality improvement activities include: social or scientific value from the quality improvement activity; scientifically valid methodology; fair participant selection to achieve a fair distribution of burdens and benefits; favorable risk-benefit, limiting risks and maximizing benefits; respect for participants by respecting privacy and confidentiality; informed consent in minimal risk quality improvement activities as part of a patient's consent for treatment; and independent review of the ethical conduct and accountability of the quality improvement activity (Lynn, J., et. al. "The Ethics of Using Quality Improvement Methods in Health Care." *Annals of Internal Medicine.* Vol. 146, Issue 9: 666–673. 2007).

Healthcare executives, in collaboration with quality improvement officers and clinical and ethics leadership, should develop a system-oriented approach and process that ensures quality improvement activities are planned and implemented in accordance with ethical standards. Ethics committees can potentially not only serve as resources to clinicians and executives planning and implementing quality improvement programs, they also can foster such efforts.

For example, an ethics committee could develop a system-wide program to ensure that a greater number of patients have documented discussions regarding end-of-life decisions. The program could include quality improvement measures to assess compliance and an increase in advance care documents. This effort would further the ethical principle of patient self-determination and the patient-centered dimension of quality care and efficiency by decreasing unwanted treatments.

Quality care is a patient expectation and a responsibility of clinicians and executives in today's healthcare organizations. Understanding the relationship between quality and ethics can strengthen efforts to provide safe, high-quality care in an ethical manner. Such an understanding will allow for providers and executives to see the synergy between quality improvement efforts and ethics initiatives. Ethics is both the foundation for quality healthcare and a driver for achieving the desired result—quality healthcare.

September/October 2008

Editor's Note: Research for this article was supported in part by the Veterans' Rural Health Initiative at the White River Junction (Vt.) VAMC. The views expressed do not represent the U.S. government or the Department of Veterans Affairs.

Addressing Compassion Fatigue

Paul B. Hofmann, DrPH, FACHE

COMPASSION FATIGUE IS an inability or reduced capacity to feel and convey genuine understanding, empathy and support. Few healthcare professionals are immune to compassion fatigue. It occurs most often when the need for compassion is great and seemingly unrelenting. In healthcare facilities, this problem usually exists when the level of stress is high, demand for attention is rising and emotional reserves appear insufficient to accommodate the needs of not only patients and families but also staff.

In the past, but presumably less so today, the very nature of medical education was blamed for dehumanizing altruistic, sensitive medical students and producing cold, impersonal and unsympathetic physicians. Some suggested it was essential the physician-patient relationship be kept as objective and formal as possible to maintain a professional rapport. Proponents of this approach said preserving a proper distance would protect physicians from becoming too vulnerable and emotionally involved with their patients.

There are, of course, other more prevalent factors leading to compassion fatigue among healthcare workers. They include lack of early encouragement from family to give and accept compassion; inadequate professional training; poor mentoring; low staffing; and an organizational culture that does not encourage, value and recognize exemplary displays of compassion.

Unquestionably, disruptive behavior of physicians, nurses, managers and others is another factor contributing to reduced compassion. Anyone who has been regularly berated and verbally abused will have a more difficult time compartmentalizing the resulting feelings and conveying compassion to patients, families and colleagues.

We know inconsiderate behavior by physicians and managers makes their subordinates' work more stressful. More specifically, if employees do not believe they are respected and appreciated for their efforts, and if they do not feel cared about by those who have responsibility for them, it will be more difficult for them to establish and sustain a truly caring environment for patients.

Also, in healthcare organizations that focus too narrowly on the achievement of standard measures, some staff members may concentrate exclusively on task completion as the goal rather than *how* the care is provided.

A colleague described a recent case where a Buddhist patient in the ICU suffered a prolonged and uncomfortable death. The patient's family had stood watch as the patient's condition deteriorated. After his death, when family members asked, based on cultural practices, if the body could lay undisturbed for a number of hours before being moved, the charge nurse denied the request.

The family members were told they had 15 minutes with their loved one because a patient in the emergency department needed the bed. In this situation, rather than working creatively to find another option that would meet the family's needs, the charge nurse focused only on the task at hand—prepare the ICU bed for the emergency department patient.

COSTS OF COMPASSION FATIGUE

In addition to patients and families, victims of compassion fatigue include clinical staff. Even nonclinical personnel, however, will be affected when workload exceeds capacity and personal and professional issues compromise normal coping techniques. Inevitably, compassion fatigue will have an adverse impact on staff recruitment, retention, morale and performance.

Predictably, those who are psychologically and physically exhausted will be less likely to show compassion. And unfortunately, in times of staff reductions and a struggling economy, the need for more compassion increases just when emotional reservoirs are lower.

According to a physician quoted in a Feb. 6, 2009, *New York Times* article, doctors and nurses "feel trapped by the competing demands of administrators, insurance companies, lawyers, patients' families and even one another." There are no signs the intensity of these demands will diminish in the near future, so we must think creatively about how to confront them successfully.

ADDRESSING COMPASSION FATIGUE

Determine whether compassion fatigue is a valid concern within your organization, and involve your staff in preparing an action plan to eliminate it if possible or at least reduce it.

Recognize and celebrate uncommon displays of compassion to indicate that such behavior is genuinely appreciated and valued.

Consider job-sharing arrangements to allow personnel in particularly stressful positions to work in other settings as well. For example, in one health system, hospice social workers and nurses work one or two days a week in another area.

Identify specific ethical issues that create moral distress (when a person knows what is ethically appropriate but is unable to act appropriately because of various obstacles). Provide opportunities to discuss how these issues can be addressed more candidly and productively.

Include nurses in discussions when physicians talk to patients about serious medical mistakes. In a study published in the January 2009 issue of *The Joint Commission Journal on Quality and Patient Safety*, the authors reported that leaving nurses out of the disclosure process may contribute to moral distress, less job satisfaction and increased turnover.

Make site visits to organizations that have won national recognition for their high patient- and staff-satisfaction rates, low nursing-vacancy rates and exceptional clinical outcomes to learn how their organizational culture has succeeded in designing and maintaining best practices.

Encourage retreats and educational opportunities that can refresh and inspire staff members to focus on compassionate care of others *and* one's self.

No healthcare executive or other healthcare professional intentionally avoids taking active steps to reduce the incidence of compassion fatigue. However, we must not ignore the high costs associated with compassion fatigue, both in terms of quality of care and financial impact. These costs may not be easy to measure precisely, but we need not wait for more definitive analyses to appreciate their ramifications.

Ideally, compassion should be demonstrated regularly and consistently. When Thomas M. Tierney was director of the Social Security Administration's bureau of health insurance more than 25 years ago he said, "law cannot create values or commitment, conscience cannot be legislated and compassion cannot be purchased." His sentiments are still valid today. Our challenge is to make certain these priceless virtues are present in all our institutions.

September/October 2009

Part IV:
An Organization's
Ethics Resources

THIS SECTION CONTAINS ethics columns that focus on an organization's various resources for addressing ethical issues. The most common ethics resource in today's healthcare facilities is an ethics committee. Because of the importance of having a competent, available, and respected ethics committee or program, *Healthcare Executive*'s Healthcare Management Ethics columns explore a number of strategies to ensure that appropriate and effective institutional resources are accessible to assist healthcare executives and other staff.

Appointing an Ethics Officer

Edward Petry, PhD

As my organization grows increasingly complex, so do the ethical dilemmas we face. Would appointing an ethics officer help us clarify these issues? What responsibilities would be inherent to this position?

In response to heightened government scrutiny, increasing application of the False Claims Act, and widespread publicity given to scandals and investigations, many healthcare organizations today are asking these questions. Increasingly, they are concluding that they need to review their internal ethics initiatives and appoint an executive to manage these programs.

Responsibilities of an ethics officer generally include managing internal reporting systems, assessing ethics risk areas, developing and distributing ethics policies and publications, investigating alleged violations, and designing training programs. Because ethics and compliance programs have similar foundations, in some organizations the ethics officer might manage compliance functions as well.

Because these responsibilities are far-reaching, this position should be primarily a management one and not just a policing and/or legal function. While ethics officers are often highly placed in the organization, the officer and the ethics program must also be backed up by other senior managers.

Smaller, single-facility healthcare organizations may be able to manage their ethics programs as a function of the human resources division. However, given the complexity of ethical dilemmas encountered in today's healthcare environment and the seriousness of the consequences if violations do occur, large, multi-site systems would be well-served by appointing an ethics officer.

If your organization chooses to do so, be aware that partial measures are not enough. Too often, a large, complex organization believes that by appointing a part-time, mid-level ethics officer, it will be able to address any ethical concerns that develop. Increasingly, however, such efforts are being viewed with suspicion. In a recent survey of Ethics Officer Association members, who represent more than 30 U.S. industries, part-time ethics officers reported an average of 96 annual contacts, including questions about policies as well as allegations of wrongdoing; full-time ethics officers, however, reported an average of 1,486 annual contacts. Some of this disparity might exist because employees believe part-time programs indicate a lack of organizational commitment to ethics. More wholehearted efforts, however, can help communicate an organization's dedication to ethical practices. In fact, a recent study by Walker Information found that when organizations provide ethics information resources such as a code of ethics, a value statement, and/or an ethics officer, employees rate them as highly ethical.

Today, every organization needs to examine its level of commitment to internal ethics by asking the following: Are we keeping up with the ethical standards of our field? Do we have a plan to keep pace with the rising expectations of the public, employees, and regulators? Are we providing adequate resources, guidance, and support to help our employees make difficult ethical decisions? Would an employee know where to turn in our organization to get help with an ethical dilemma? Would they be willing to report a possible violation without fear of retaliation? And most importantly, are we taking all necessary steps to prevent and detect violation of law, regulations, and corporate policies? If the answer to any of these questions is no, consider learning from other organizations who have already been down this road.

November/December 1995

Evaluating Your Ethics Committees

William A. Nelson, PhD

As the CEO of a mid-sized medical center, how can I be assured that our organization's ethics committee is effective and capable of serving as a useful resource to our clinicians and administration?

The importance, goals, and functions of healthcare ethics committees are clearly evolving in relation to the changing healthcare environment. Historically, ethics committees have been acute-care oriented, often confronting ethical medical dilemmas related to the end of life. Today, healthcare organizations are becoming increasingly primary care and outpatient focused—and the distinction between bedside and boardroom ethical issues is becoming increasingly blurred. In response, ethics committees are being required to widen their scope to include clinical and organizational ethics alike. In an era of managed care, ethics committees must be capable of addressing such issues as the allocation of hospital resources or the role of clinicians as gatekeepers. In other words, they must confront broader mission, policy, and procedural concerns, not just individual patient issues.

As the complexity and urgency of ethical healthcare issues escalate, your organization may increasingly turn to its ethics committee for guidance and direction. To determine if your ethics committee is positioned to act effectively, review the following dimensions of your committee.

PURPOSE AND FUNCTIONS

All ethics committee members, as well as your organization's staff and administration, should understand and accept the purpose and functions of the committee. To evaluate how clearly the ethics committee's purpose is defined, ask committee members to answer this question: "What is the purpose of our committee?" This question often elicits surprisingly different responses, even if the group has been working together for several years. Before gaining organizationwide support, you must achieve consensus within the committee as to its purpose and goals.

Once the committee's purpose is defined and accepted, establish clear guidelines regarding how the ethics committee performs its functions, including policy review, education, evaluation, and clinical/organizational ethics consultations. For example, how will the committee carry out its ethics consultations? Does the whole committee consult on an issue, or does a smaller team respond? Who on the committee does staff contact with ethical concerns? To determine how informed your staff is about your ethics committee, ask individuals in various departments how they would access the ethics committee and what they would expect to accomplish by consulting it. You may discover that you need to educate staff about the ethics committee's purpose and processes so that its potential as an internal resource is maximized. Without clarity and acceptance of purpose, functions, and structure, your ethics committee may not be perceived as a useful resource.

COMPOSITION AND COMPETENCIES OF MEMBERS

Broad and balanced professional representation is essential for your committee to be respected and used by your staff and administration. Because cultural perspective influences how people approach illness, ethics committee membership should reflect the diversity of the healthcare organization and the community it serves. For example, if a dominant religious or ethnic population is being served by your organization, those communities must be represented by the ethics committee membership. Furthermore, to ensure active participation by its members, ethics committees should be composed primarily of volunteers, rather than individuals who are assigned to serve on the committee. Recruit new members by identifying individuals in your organization who show interest and demonstrate reasoned thinking regarding ethical issues. Survey staff and co-workers, and take note of those who participate in common educational activities that pertain to ethical issues.

In addition to possessing interest, motivation, and time, the best ethics committee members will be those who possess a comprehensive set of competencies. The American Society for Bioethics and Humanities' 1998 report, "Core Competencies for Health Care Ethics Consultation," offers guidelines for the appropriate knowledge, skills, and character for those performing ethics consultations. The report identifies three major skill sets:

- **Ethical assessment skills** enable individuals to identify the values underlying ethical conflicts. These skills include the ability to distinguish the ethical dimensions of a situation from other overlapping dimensions, such as legal or medical; to access, critically evaluate, and use relevant knowledge; to identify and justify various morally acceptable options and their consequences; and to evaluate evidence and arguments for and against different solutions.
- **Process skills** focus on efforts to resolve the uncertainty related to values that arises in healthcare settings. These skills include the ability to facilitate meetings, identify key decision makers, create an atmosphere of trust, negotiate between competing moral views, and engage in creative problem solving.
- **Interpersonal skills** include the ability to listen effectively, educate concerned parties about the ethical dimensions of their dilemma, and represent the views of concerned parties to others.

In addition to these general skills, the ASBH identified nine core knowledge areas that are required for competent ethical consultation. Your ethics committee should be populated by individuals who possess some level of knowledge in these areas, which include an understanding of the following:

- Moral reasoning and ethical theory
- Common bioethical issues and concepts
- Healthcare systems, which includes knowledge of managed care and governmental systems
- Clinical context
- Your healthcare organization, including the organization's mission statement and structure
- Your healthcare organization's policies
- Beliefs and perspectives of the local patient and staff population
- Relevant codes of ethics and professional conduct and guidelines of accrediting organizations
- Relevant health law

In addition to this knowledge, ethics consultants—similar to all healthcare professionals—should possess and exhibit good character, which includes tolerance, honesty, courage, prudence, and integrity.

LEADERSHIP

The chairperson of your ethics committee must be well respected within your organization, have a comprehensive understanding of the organization's formal and informal decision-making processes, and be open to input and feedback from committee members and staff. To keep your ethics committee viable and dynamic, the chairperson should not be a "fixture"; in other words, he or she should not hold the position to the point where the committee becomes dependent on that individual. The committee should be structured so that all members actively contribute and tasks are fairly distributed.

ORGANIZATIONAL SUPPORT AND RESPECT

To ensure quality in the functions of the ethics committee, your organization must support and respect its role. Administration and trustees should help ethics committee members develop competencies by providing educational resources and ensuring that members are given adequate time for their ethics committee duties. Furthermore, it is crucial that the organization create a climate for the committee to carry out its activities with integrity. The committee should not be expected to simply echo the organization's position on certain issues; rather, they must be able to speak freely in an appropriate and tactful manner, regardless of the organization's stance. Only then will honest dialogue take place between the administration and the committee to enhance the overall ethical nature of the organization.

Ethics committees that are well informed, representative, and motivated can be a healthcare organization's greatest resource for ethical guidance and support.

January/February 2000

Improving Ethics Committee Effectiveness

Paul B. Hofmann, DrPH, FACHE

We have a well-organized ethics committee that has produced useful policies, consulted on cases, and sponsored education programs for both the staff and the community. Nonetheless, case consultation requests are rare, and we feel that the committee's resources in other areas are not used to their potential. What should we do?

Your concerns are not uncommon. Many ethics committees are struggling with their role, confused about their responsibilities beyond the traditional focus on clinical issues. The rising interest in organizational, business, and management ethics, along with corporate compliance, has prompted ethics committees to reassess their goals and objectives.

When hospital executives were asked at an ACHE seminar (in 2000) if the ethics committees in their organizations were highly effective, very few individuals replied affirmatively. Consequently, it is not surprising that committee members may be questioning their value to the organization.

POSSIBLE REASONS FOR UNDERUTILIZATION

Your staff may not be making the most of your ethics committee for a variety of reasons. Among them are:

- **Inaccurate understanding of the committee's role and potential contribution.** Some staff members may think the committee's sole function is to provide case consultation when there is concern about an end-of-life dilemma. Others may hesitate to ask for assistance because they do not want to be obligated to comply with the ethics committee's conclusion, failing to realize that the committee is an advisory, not a decision-making, body. Still others may be concerned about conveying extremely sensitive information, not recognizing the committee's efforts to preserve nondisclosure and confidentiality.
- **Low visibility.** Depending on the location of your committee in your organizational structure, publicity about its purpose, and periodic reports on its activity, many people may be unaware of its existence and the resource it represents.
- **Uncertainty about how to gain access to the committee.** If your committee has a low organizational profile, and there is no convenient way to contact a committee representative and receive a timely response, it is understandable why few requests for assistance are received.
- **Inadequate committee representation.** The size, diversity (including cultural and religious), and number of disciplines represented on your committee will certainly be related to your organization's size and mission, but the group should not be composed only of physicians and nurses. Restricting the membership in this way can bias perceptions of the committee's insight, credibility, and objectivity.
- **Ineffectual leadership.** As is true of any committee, the effectiveness of your ethics committee will often be directly related to the ability of its chairperson. Obviously, if this individual is

disorganized, autocratic, or ingenuous, there will be fewer requests for consultation and other assistance.

- **Insufficient organizational support.** Although major funding is not required to facilitate a committee's activities, there must be a reasonable budget to cover the cost of publications and similar resources to support the continuing education of both committee members and stakeholders.
- **Lack of initiative.** A failure to develop and implement a creative strategic plan could be the most prevalent reason an ethics committee is underused and, as a result, marginally effective. Too many committees are simply passive and reactive, instead of pursuing a formal set of goals and objectives to maximize their value to the organizations they serve.

PRACTICAL STRATEGIES

To address your concern, you should first ask the committee to complete a comprehensive assessment of its performance. Such an audit should review the committee's purpose, composition, and activities. Begin by asking committee members to provide their assessment of the committee's:

1. Vision, values, and scope of services
2. Structure, authority, and relationship with other organizational entities
3. Frequency, convenience, and length of meetings; adequacy of agenda; and educational material
4. Process for evaluating its accomplishments, strengths, and weaknesses; communications within and outside the organization; effectiveness of its policies and guidelines; and customer feedback
5. Success in defining and addressing its educational needs and those of the hospital community

6. Development, revision, and impact of ethical policies and guidelines
7. Resource support requirements
8. Case consultation process

After this self-assessment survey is completed and tabulated, you should share and discuss the results at the committee's annual retreat. It is likely that the group's annual goals and objectives will include preparing an action plan to address issues highlighted in the responses. Organizationwide surveys of past and potential committee users can also prove effective.

As mentioned, some committees have been asked to examine organizational ethics, and your committee could easily review the growing literature on this topic and initiate appropriate proposals or programs. Such an initiative might involve changing the scope of committee activities, its composition, and other aspects of its operation. Even if the number and magnitude of changes are relatively small, the organization, its staff, and patients will be the ultimate beneficiaries of a revitalized committee.

January/February 2001

The practical strategies for the committee self-assessment come from Rebecca Dobbs's doctoral dissertation, which was recently submitted to Walden University in Minneapolis, MN.

Responding to Unusual Ethical Dilemmas

Paul B. Hofmann, DrPH, FACHE

Recently, our hospital was approached by a family member who asked that sperm be obtained from a relative who was a deceased patient. We have no policy for such a request, so it was denied. Is there a model policy dealing with this issue?

Over time, a healthcare organization will encounter a variety of dilemmas with ethical implications for patients, family members, and staff. In addition to the example above, there have been cases involving the adequacy of informed consent, a patient's decision-making capacity, abusive patients and family members, the HIV/AIDS status of a patient or staff member, preferential treatment of benefactors, patient and staff confidentiality, and myriad other issues, many of which are neither preventable nor predictable. One way to address such issues is to create a new policy each time a unique situation occurs. A more practical alternative is to develop a generic policy that will serve several purposes:

- Acknowledging that many dilemmas cannot be foreseen but do deserve a thoughtful response when they arise.

- Providing a process for accommodating unprecedented events, thus increasing the likelihood that responses will be consistent, rational, and timely.
- Reminding medical staff members and others that the ethics committee (or whatever mechanism the organization has adopted to address ethical issues, e.g., ethics consultation service) is a valuable and useful organizational resource.

Perhaps most important, careful deliberation of how unusual dilemmas should be addressed will require a reflection of the organization's values. If the generic policy is properly crafted, subsequent decisions should be compatible with these values.

CONTENT AREAS FOR POLICY

When crafting a generic ethical policy, you will want to include the following elements:

1. **A preface.** A preface should describe both the policy's purpose and the importance of its consistent application to ensure that the organization's values are considered in addressing unanticipated ethical dilemmas.
2. **A list of potential resources.** Organizational resources that may be used to address an issue should be identified, e.g., administration, human resources, risk management, legal counsel, ethics committee, ethics consultant, public/community relations, social services, chaplain's office. By preparing a comprehensive checklist, you could avoid inadvertently overlooking an important ally.
3. **A review of procedures.** Procedures should be listed that promote a rapid, confidential, and effective resolution of the dilemma. Such procedures include: when and how to report the issue; to whom the report should be made; measures to

maintain confidentiality; guidelines for responding to potential media requests; the process to be followed to achieve closure; and steps to prevent, minimize, or more adequately resolve similar dilemmas in the future.

Depending upon the nature of the dilemma and its possible ramifications, there may be a role for the executive committee of the medical staff or board of trustees. Alternatively, it may suffice to involve or inform the medical staff president and/or the board chair. Inevitably, requests or issues will arise that will suggest the need to revise or refine the generic policy, but this policy should be no different than the others, which should also be reviewed periodically to confirm their continuing validity and relevancy.

OTHER CONSIDERATIONS

Too often, organizations neglect an essential step in maintaining and advancing their ethical sensitivity in today's increasingly complex healthcare environment, namely, conducting a prompt and complete evaluation of a specific request or incident. This step might include a formal audit of the organization's response and the subsequent results. You might find that, in retrospect,

- communication could have been handled differently;
- there were too few or too many participants involved in handling the issue;
- the situation could have been resolved more quickly;
- there were other steps that could have prevented the issue or conflict from escalating;
- economic factors had too little or too much influence on the outcome; or
- other options might have been more effective in satisfying the needs of the patient, family, and/or staff members.

It is neither realistic nor productive for organizations to consider the development of policies covering every ethical dilemma. However, organizations should develop a generic policy that provides general guidelines for responding to exceptional requests and conflicts. Patients and their families, as well as physicians and employees, will be the ultimate beneficiaries.

July/August 2002

The Value of an Ethics Audit

Paul B. Hofmann, DrPH, FACHE

*Like most organizations, we have well-crafted vision, mission and val-
ues statements, but it is difficult to determine our compliance with these
statements. Is there a tool or process that can help us take our ethical pulse?*

An ethics audit is a practical and valuable tool to evaluate where
the organization may be falling below its own standards and expectations. Such an audit involves a comprehensive review of policies,
procedures and perceptions to determine consistency with the organization's vision, mission, and values. When conducted properly, it
provides an excellent snapshot of the institution's ethical climate.

The audit helps identify real and perceived problems. Both types
of problems must be recognized to address them effectively. However,
similar to performing any survey, it creates expectations that the
findings will be summarized and shared, and an action plan will be
prepared and implemented to deal with deficiencies.

SYMPTOMS SUGGESTING THE NEED FOR AN AUDIT

Employees, physicians and even communities are aware when an
organization's rhetoric does not match reality. To avoid professional

hypocrisy, practices must not contradict the institution's proclamations. A number of factors may suggest that an ethics audit should be initiated. These factors include

- decline in patient, employee or physician satisfaction ratings;
- higher turnover rates;
- reduction in community support as evidenced by the number and size of donations, number of volunteers and average weekly hours, and attendance at sponsored programs/events;
- allegations of conflicts of interest; or
- increase in litigation against the institution.

Ironically, the most important of these is none of the above. Indeed, an ideal time to perform an ethics audit is when there is no crisis or compelling set of problems. Every organization can benefit by periodically evaluating its ethical behavior.

AHA ORGANIZATIONAL ETHICS INITIATIVE

Ten years ago, as a member of the American Hospital Association's Organizational Ethics Task Force, I suggested the development of an ethics audit. Working with the assistance of the Ethics Resource Center in Washington, DC, the task force produced a six-part organizational assessment tool. The six parts, which remain relevant today, focus on the following:

- Part one focused on existing organizational materials and raised questions about written statements of ethical principles, codes of conduct and pertinent policies and procedures. For example, what procedures help assure compliance with ethical requirements?
- Part two dealt with training, publications, and formal processes. For example, what would an employee be expected

to do if he or she became aware of unethical activity and what steps would the organization take in responding to the report?

- Part three inquired about organizational structure. For example, if an ethics committee exists, what is its role in organizational ethics?
- Part four raised questions about organizational character. For example, what are the institution's ethical obligations to its community?
- Part five elicited the most significant ethical challenges facing the organization; respondents to a questionnaire were asked to rank, in order of priority, 24 potential issues.
- Part six was a survey that asked employees to assess the organization's ethics standards and practices; staff members were asked to indicate their degree of agreement or disagreement with 55 statements.

CONDUCTING AN ETHICS AUDIT AND BENEFITING FROM ITS RESULTS

As noted previously, an ethics audit should not be undertaken unless management is genuinely interested in sharing and addressing the findings. Once the commitment has been confirmed, a plan should be developed that provides a specific timeline for each component. These components include preparing a communication strategy to inform the organization and its stakeholders of the audit; collecting and analyzing appropriate documents; reviewing roles and responsibilities of key staff members and relevant committees; preparing interview and survey documents; performing the interviews and conducting the surveys; determining where there are contradictions and inconsistencies; and compiling and disseminating the results.

Of course, now comes the most critical step—after a complete diagnostic picture has been taken, detailed plans must be developed to address problem areas. Such plans might include redesigning interview and employment procedures. For instance, some employers ask about an applicant's values, describe those of the organization, and obtain a commitment from the applicant to support them.

Other steps could involve redesigning orientation and in-service education programs; establishing new policies, positions or committees; revising existing position descriptions or committee responsibilities; creating a casebook on ethical dilemmas for use in supervisory training to assist them in recognizing and reconciling competing values; implementing a telephone hotline to report questionable conduct; expanding the role of the institution's ethics committee to cover issues relating to both organizational and clinical ethics; and re-emphasizing compliance with the organization's code of conduct during performance reviews.

An ethics audit can be a powerful tool to acquire fresh insights about any major business. In a healthcare setting, if undertaken carefully, the ultimate beneficiaries should be patients and their families as well as the organization itself.

March/April 2006

Defining Ethics

William A. Nelson, PhD

We have an active ethics committee that addresses ethical conflicts and questions. What is an "ethical" conflict, and what type of situation might warrant a consultation with the ethics committee?

Just as ethics committees should have an established set of guidelines, including their purpose and functions as they have been approved by the leadership and shared throughout the organization, ethics committee members ought to have an agreed-upon understanding of what constitutes an ethical conflict and is appropriate for their review.

Clinicians and administrators regularly confront a wide variety of conflicts or uncertainty regarding the best action to take or the right decision to implement. However, those conflicts are not necessarily *ethical* in nature but rather are legal, financial, administrative, or clinical conflicts.

The classic definition of an ethical conflict is when a person—or an institution acting as a moral agent—is considering violating a moral principle or rule (a commonly accepted ethical norm), such as "do not deceive" or "do not deprive freedom." This definition of ethical conflicts also includes instances when a conflict or uncertainty arises between competing, commonly accepted moral principles, as well as established professional or organizational ethics standards. A healthcare ethics conflict, by its nature, is a situation that seems to elude obvious resolution, that is, one's moral intuition. No morally right or good options clearly present themselves because alternatives to the conflict carry both good and bad elements.

To illustrate this definition, consider a patient safety officer who encounters many conflicts requiring a decision. All those conflicts are not of an ethical nature. The patient safety officer may need to choose among several competing software products to track patient safety encounters. Deciding what software to purchase is challenging and may require the perspective of a consultant to assist in deciding which software is best given the established norms, such as budget, user friendliness, and compatibility with the current computer system.

The uncertainty involved in choosing the right software for the facility does not necessarily constitute an ethical conflict because the conflict or uncertainty is not related to competing ethical principles or rules. The conflict is over which product best meets technical or practical standards. However, the decision of what software to purchase can become an ethical conflict if the patient safety officer decides to purchase a software package that costs significantly more than the allotted budget and he or she does not intend to inform the leadership of the cost overrun. In such a situation the officer is considering violating the general moral rule of "do not deceive." The same moral rule is the foundation for proactively developing organizational guidelines requiring disclosure of adverse events to patients or their representative.

Another ethical conflict would occur if the patient safety officer is considering taking a vendor's offer of a trip to a Florida resort to discuss its software product. This is an ethical conflict for the patient safety officer because he or she is considering violating the organization and the profession's (ACHE) code of ethics concerning conflicts of interest.

The various definitions of an ethical conflict are linked to an understanding of what is ethics, which is a general term for seeking to determine what is morally right or wrong—what a person or institution should or should not do morally when values compete or conflict. Approaches to determining what one ought to do in a given conflict include applying and ranking normative ethical standards or principles that emanate from various ethical theories. The ethical theories seek to promote clarity, systematic reasoning, and comprehensive inquiry regarding the application of moral standards.

Because moral principles are general, various professional organizations, including those of healthcare executives, physicians, and nurses, have developed more specific ethical standards to guide the behavior of members of their particular profession. Specific ethical standards, such as the American College of Healthcare Executives' *Code of Ethics*, are derived from the more general, commonly accepted moral principles. For example, autonomy, or "do not deprive freedom," in the context of healthcare fosters the moral standard of obtaining the patient's valid informed consent or refusal prior to treatment.

Such specific ethics guidelines are frequently referred to as professional ethics. They do not replace the general principles but make ethical behavior more specific for a particular group. Therefore, ethical conflicts can result from conflicts between or uncertainty about the general moral standards as well as the more specific professional ethics.

In the second part of your question you seek clarification about when someone should seek an ethics consultation regarding an ethical conflict. Ethics committee protocols vary from organization to organization, but generally it would be appropriate for anyone in the organization to seek the perspective of the ethics committee when the parties involved in the conflict are uncertain about what to do or how to apply the commonly accepted moral principles or the organization's more specific established ethics guidelines.

July/August 2006

Dealing with Ethical Challenges

William A. Nelson, PhD

Ethical conflicts can be detrimental to the organization. Are there ways to decrease the frequency of ethical conflicts?

Ethical challenges are a common occurrence for both clinicians and healthcare executives. Many hospitals and other healthcare organizations have ethics committees to help clinicians and administrators respond to ethical conflicts or questions. Ethics committees have a long history; however, the past 10–15 years have seen a shift in the scope, reach and responsibilities of the traditional ethics committee. The shift includes:

- focusing on today's expanded healthcare delivery environment to include outpatient and primary care settings, as well as the inpatient setting;
- addressing organizational and management issues in addition to clinical conflicts;
- directing activities toward the organization's mission, code of ethics, and value statement, not just individual patient rights;
- applying a proactive approach in addition to a reactive approach to ethical conflicts;

- establishing clinical and administrative ethical practice guidelines or protocols;
- being accountable according to measurable quality improvement outcomes;
- increasing the competency and diversity of ethics committee membership; and
- being an organizationally integrated committee, including linkages to administrative leadership and other programs and committees rather than a segregated "silo."

These changes reflect a growing recognition of the organization's current ethics needs and the importance of ethics to its success. The shift also reflects the perspective that ethical practices are linked to the overall quality of care provided by the organization.

The shift from a more traditional model varies significantly among facilities. Variations in the scope, effectiveness and integration of the ethics committee into the organization are dependent on the executive's belief in the importance of ethics to the organization's mission.

Perhaps the most important of these new trends has been the evolution to a more proactive or preventive approach to dealing with ethical issues. Since their inception, a common activity for ethics committees is to provide a consultation service to assist staff in addressing ethical conflicts. This approach tends to be in response to an existing, immediate conflict. This traditional reactive approach to complex and challenging ethical conflicts can be helpful to the involved parties. However, using the traditional process has several potential concerns.

Responding to an ethical conflict can be stressful and carry time limitations that can affect a thoughtful assessment of the conflict. The presence of ethical conflicts can potentially take a toll on the culture of the organization and the involved staff because of the inherent uncertainty surrounding the conflict. It also has been suggested that a traditional approach tends to accept that ethical conflicts are recurring while ignoring the underlining system or organizational structure causing the conflict. Despite these concerns, having a competent and available ethics consultation program is essential because ethical conflicts will arise and need immediate attention.

ADOPTING A PROACTIVE APPROACH

What may be an arguably more important feature of an ethics committee is having a proactive approach to ethical conflicts. A proactive approach, emphasizing the prevention of ethical conflicts by fostering the development of ethical practice protocols or guidelines that are integrated into the culture of the organization, can enhance the quality of care and is a way to reduce the frequency of ethical conflicts.

The proactive approach to addressing ethical conflicts is based on five basic steps:

1. Identify the recurring ethical issues that create conflict or uncertainty.
2. Study the ethical issues in a systematic and system-oriented manner.
3. Develop ethical practice protocols to guide clinicians and executives when the conflict arises again.
4. Propagate the protocols into the organization's culture so all staff are aware of the guidelines and the rationale driving the guidance.
5. Review whether the protocols are adequately addressing and decreasing the occurrence of the ethical conflicts.

The proactive, preventive approach can be used in various settings and situations. For example, a member of the ethics committee could meet with the patient safety officer, head of human resources, vice president of operations or the intensive care staff and ask, "What are the recurring ethical issues you and your staff encounter?"

Those identified and prioritized ethical issues could be systematically and thoughtfully discussed with all appropriate parties leading to an ethically grounded, proactive set of guidelines. Once the guidelines are shared, the level of uncertainty can be decreased.

Another situation where a proactive approach could be employed is when the ethics committee members recognize that cases brought to their attention raise a recurring ethical issue. The recognition that ethical cases recur strongly suggests that guidelines are needed.

Even though a thoughtful process leading to the development of a set of ethical guidelines may seem time consuming and arduous, it has the advantage of creating an environment of increased ethical certainty and staff satisfaction by avoiding stressful ethical conflicts. In the long run, the preventive approach will decrease the ethical conflicts from escalating into troubling issues for the staff.

Despite the importance of developing a proactive approach, ethics committees should continue to have a competent and available reactive ethics case consultation service to address clinical and organizational ethics questions that require an immediate response. However, the addition of a preventive approach also is needed. The approach will enhance the organization's overall ethical culture by helping staff understand the right thing to do, thus reducing the occurrence of ethical conflicts.

March/April 2007

Ethics Programs in
Small Rural Hospitals

William A. Nelson, PhD

I am CEO of a rural critical-access hospital (CAH), and we currently do not have an ethics committee. What approaches should we take in the development of an ethics committee?

Ethics committees are an important resource for addressing ethical conflicts for healthcare providers and administrators in all healthcare facilities. Even though ethics committees have evolved throughout the past few decades, there is a generally accepted purpose, structure, and set of functions framing the traditional ethics committee. The basic functions include ethics education, institutional policy review and development, and case consultation. The focus of these activities is primarily clinical, with some committees also addressing organizational ethics conflicts. Ethics committees vary in effectiveness, structure and function, though they tend to include multidisciplinary professionals and have defined functions and processes, regular meetings, member participation in meetings, consultation services, ethics education, and a trained ethics expert available to advise and educate members.

Unlike their large, urban counterparts, small, rural healthcare facilities are less likely to have ethics committees. Survey data from various regions have suggested that approximately 50 percent of small, rural hospitals have ethics committees or programs for providing ethics services. Where rural ethics committees exist, however, they do not always conform to the traditional structure.

Obstacles are frequently encountered when establishing or maintaining an ethics committee in rural CAHs. One obstacle is the lack of multidisciplinary professionals found in rural CAHs. Small, rural hospitals tend to have limited services and diversity of healthcare professionals, such as mental health professionals, which reduces the possibility of having a multidisciplinary committee. A second obstacle is that many members of rural ethics committees lack ethics training, and there are few rural ethics case consultants with the recommended knowledge and skills for performing consultations. When ethics training and resources are sought, the content rarely focuses on ethics conflicts occurring within rural contexts. A third obstacle is lack of a regulatory requirement for an ethics "mechanism." Rural hospitals are less likely than urban facilities to be reviewed by The Joint Commission, which requires an ethics mechanism to address ethics conflicts. A fourth obstacle is because of the small size of rural communities, overlapping and dual relationships are common. For example, the nurse chair of the ethics committee may be responding to an ethical conflict focusing on a neighbor or former church/school teacher, which raises interpersonal dynamic challenges rarely seen in urban facilities. A fifth and final obstacle is that the small staffs of CAHs have little time to participate on a committee, and the facility has limited economic resources to support the committee.

Despite these and other obstacles, the availability of an ethics committee is important for both clinicians and administrators to ensure quality healthcare by addressing ethical challenges; therefore, rural facility leadership should employ the following strategies to help ensure there is a competent and effective mechanism to address ethics conflicts in their organizations:

- The administrative leadership and governing board need to recognize the importance of ethics and an ethics committee.

Because effective ethics committees can enhance the quality of care by fostering ethical practices and reducing stressful, time-consuming ethical conflicts, ethics committees need to be seen as essential to organizations. Rather than being an economic burden, ethics committees can be economically beneficial to the organization. However, without complete administrative support it is unlikely that an effective committee will be created and sustained.

- Facility leaders should appoint a chair of their ethics committee and support them in the development of their ethics-related knowledge and skills. The primary criterion for the chair includes an interest in ethics, organizational respect, willingness to develop their ethics knowledge and skills, and the ability to dedicate time specifically for ethics. The ethics chair can guide the committee's activities, including selecting a diverse, multi-disciplinary group of professionals to join the committee. Community representatives, such as clergy and board members, can augment the available healthcare professionals.

- Rural ethics committees can be linked to statewide ethics networks, which can foster useful support for often isolated rural committees. State ethics network meetings can enhance rural ethics committee members' knowledge. Rural committee members should encourage network coordinators to regularly address ethical issues unique to rural committees.

- Rural ethics committees should make contact with academic-based ethics centers. Even though many centers focus on issues that relate to the needs of large, academic and metropolitan communities, there is a growing understanding and awareness of rural healthcare ethics. Such contact can potentially foster the activities of the rural committee.

- The ethics committee can explore the expanding array of rural ethics literature and identify a rural focused healthcare ethicist. Through electronic and telephone consultation the rural healthcare ethicist can serve as a useful advisor or resource to the committee.

- When there are limited resources at one facility to support an ethics committee, another option is a multifacility ethics committee (MFEC). The MFEC model is particularly plausible where there is an existing set of linkages between facilities. This model has the potential to be efficient and effective by sharing ethics expertise and financial support.
- Each participating facility would identify one or two professionals to serve on the committee and then would provide financial support for its representatives and modest support for the MFEC's general operation. The support could be pooled without overly taxing any individual facility. Because of geographical distances between facilities and time restraints, regular meetings could be conducted by conference calling or, where available, video conferencing.

Ethics committees in both rural and urban healthcare facilities are an important resource for clinicians and administrators regardless of the size or location of the facility. Because the rural context is woven into the fabric of the ethical challenges encountered, having an available rural ethics committee can significantly contribute to the organization's quality of care.

There never will be one model for "doing ethics" because rural committees' activities need to be prioritized to address the facility's needs and issues. However, most committees will likely include ethics education, policy, ethics practice guideline development and case consultation. What is essential is that an organization's CEO openly supports and seeks out an active ethics committee. When this occurs, and a local ethics expert emerges, rural facilities reap the benefits.

November/December 2007

Addressing Organizational Ethics

William A. Nelson, PhD

Our organization has an effective clinical ethics committee. What advice would you offer for expanding the scope of the committee to address organizational ethical concerns?

Historically, healthcare ethics committees have focused on clinically related ethical concerns. For example, an ethics committee might provide decision-making assistance to clinical staff regarding the appropriateness of discontinuing a terminal patient's life-sustaining treatment.

More recently, healthcare ethics has expanded its focus to explore the broader organizational context of ethical uncertainties or conflicts. Organizational ethics focuses beyond individual patients to groups of people, reflecting on professional groups' (nurses, healthcare executives, etc.) ethical standards of practice or the organization's operations, policies, practices and decisions. Despite the growing interest in organizational ethics, facility decisions regarding organizational operations and practices—such as management's discussions about the development of a potentially high revenue-generating plastic surgery center rather than a community-based medical clinic in a low-income part of the community—have generally been beyond the scope of most ethics committees. Because ethical conflicts can occur in both contexts—clinical and organizational—some facilities' ethics committees recognize that they can no longer have a narrow, clinical focus regarding ethical conflicts.

THREE BASIC APPROACHES

Recognizing that both clinical and organizational ethical conflicts can affect patient care and the organization's overall practices, there is a need for ethics resources to address both. There are three basic approaches for expanding the role of the traditional clinically focused ethics committee to also address organizational ethics questions:

- One approach is to maintain the committee as it is but expand the scope of the traditional clinical-oriented committee's activities to also address organizational ethics issues. To effectively facilitate such an expanded role would require revising the committee's mission and increasing the number of committee members to include professionals from management who possess business, health policy and financial management knowledge and experience. This model has several advantages, especially in situations where the clinical committee is respected throughout the organization and its members possess the skills necessary to participate in an ethical analysis. The challenges for such a model are that the committee may be too active and too comfortable with clinical issues and that an expanded scope may be resisted. In addition, the clinically based committee members may have limited organizational and business knowledge to make the transition to addressing organizational issues.
- A second approach would be to create a new organizational ethics committee that focuses on business, financial, and other organizational ethics concerns and questions and is separate from the organization's clinical ethics committee. Members of the management team should be included in this new committee.

One advantage of this model is a dedicated group of members who possess the necessary business and administrative background and training to handle organizational ethics issues. Challenges to this model are to ensure that the members have ethics knowledge and skills to complement their business and management knowledge and determine which cases are appropriate for the clinical versus the organizational ethics committee. There may be some ethical conflicts that are clearly organizational or clinical, but this is rare and occurs because of a limited understanding of the conflict. For example, in the case of the patient who is terminal, despite being focused on an individual patient, the decisions and actions surrounding the case clearly reflect on the hospital's image and relate to the organization's policies. Therefore, a separate organizational ethics committee could prevent a clear link to the clinical ethics committee, creating confusion regarding the scope of the committee.

- A third option is to maintain one ethics committee but expand its mission and restructure it to include two subgroups: one that focuses on clinical concerns and one that focuses on organizational concerns. The advantage to this model is that it eliminates any confusion regarding which committee addresses ethical concerns. Also, the existing clinically oriented ethics committee members should possess the ethics reasoning and facilitation skills needed for exploring organizational conflicts. The committee will need to expand the membership's professional diversity to include members who work in the administrative and business aspects of healthcare. Members with healthcare business and finance training would serve as the core members of the organizational subgroup, while the clinically oriented members would focus on clinical conflicts. When ethics conflicts overlap between clinical and organizational issues, the two subgroups can collaborate. Such a collaborative process can serve as an educational vehicle to cross-fertilize the clinical and organization knowledge and skills of one subgroup with another.

I prefer the combined ethics committee because of the overlapping nature of clinical and organizational ethics concerns, the limited number of staff willing to serve on multiple committees, the challenge in trying to coordinate the activities between different committees, and the benefits of avoiding a siloed approach to ethics.

No one model or adaptation of the basic styles noted above is appropriate for all facilities. The ethics mechanism's form should be structured based on the facility's ethics committee's mission within the context of the unique environment and culture of the organization. For example, the large, urban academic medical center mechanisms for addressing clinical and organizational issues will likely look quite different from a small, rural medical center's mechanisms for addressing such issues. Yet, they will likely have similar goals: promoting the organization's mission-driven values and ethical practices throughout the organization and, ultimately, quality patient care.

What is essential in any of the models is that there is institutional leadership support and that committee members possess the appropriate knowledge and skills. To address organizational ethics questions, committee members should, in addition to having ethical reasoning skills, be knowledgeable in five fundamental areas:

- **Healthcare business practices** such as contracting and vendor relationships
- **Financial management** such as resource allocation and cost containment strategies
- **Marketing and public relations** such as the need for transparency and advertising approaches
- **Human relations** such as hiring and promoting practices
- **Community and societal obligations** such as cultural sensitivity and issues surrounding access to healthcare for the uninsured

Whatever committee or program structure seems the best option for expanding the scope of the current clinical ethics committee needs to be carefully planned and reviewed with leadership staff. Such planning includes developing a clear committee mission and defined goals and finding members who can competently address both organizational and clinical ethics challenges.

March/April 2008

An Executive-Driven
Ethical Culture

William A. Nelson, PhD, and John Donnellan, FACHE

AN ORGANIZATION'S CULTURE plays a significant role in providing an identity to staff members and shaping their behavior. The culture encompasses many elements, including shared values and beliefs, implicit and patterned assumptions that influence staff decisions, and observable characteristics such as dress, rituals, and communication. Culture is a key driver in establishing and maintaining an ethical organization because of its effect on staff members' actions.

An ethics-grounded culture needs to be a top priority for healthcare executives because of its importance to quality care and, ultimately, the organization's success overall. The culture can never be taken for granted and may need periodic renewal.

Today's healthcare executives should review, reflect, and, when needed, foster changes to their organizations' cultures. Conduct an honest, systematic review of your own executive behaviors and your organization's ethical culture. This can be done by using ACHE's Ethics Self-Assessment, available in the Ethics area of **ache.org** and once a year in *Healthcare Executive*, and by talking openly and honestly with your organization's ethics committee, senior leadership, and staff. You may be persuaded of the need for cultural change.

Improving the ethical culture is not easy, it takes time, and it will not happen by accident. It requires thoughtful, dedicated focus that actively involves healthcare leadership. There are fundamental components of an institution's culture—mission/vision/values; organizational structure, including a formal ethics program; and leadership behavior—that can address these issues and serve as building blocks for an organization's ethical framework.

MISSION, VISION, AND VALUES

A healthcare organization must begin by establishing or reviewing the statement of values upon which the organization's mission and vision are grounded. Those values must be clearly communicated to all employees early and often, beginning with the interviewing process, reinforced during employee orientation and regularly acknowledged during performance reviews, public ceremonies, celebrations, and awards. The statement of values should reflect the organization's commitment to integrity, transparency, and safety, in addition to quality and efficiency.

The mission, vision, and values cannot be simply words in a document. The document should meet the expectation of all staff members. In addition, employee position descriptions and performance evaluations need to be aligned with organizational values. For example, the organization should place an emphasis on error reporting, patient disclosure, and identification of safety vulnerabilities that is equal to the emphasis it places on achieving quality, utilization, and financial targets. Staff should be acknowledged, rewarded, and celebrated when behaviors exemplify organizational values. Leaders of healthcare organizations should consider celebrating actions taken by individuals or units that may not have achieved an intended objective but that exemplify an unwavering adherence to the organization's values.

Mission, Vision, and Values Checklist

❑ Have your mission, vision, and values been recently updated?
❑ Are all employees aware of the organization's mission, vision, and values?
❑ Are the mission, vision, and values integrated into all employees' position descriptions and performance reviews?
❑ Do clinical and administrative decisions reflect the organization's mission, vision, and values?

AN EFFECTIVE ETHICS PROGRAM

Healthcare executives must ensure that an effective formal ethics program infrastructure exists to both proactively promote ethical practices and clarify ethical uncertainty when needed. The ethics program should be system oriented and integrated into daily life at the organization.

The ethics mechanism should be available to address a broad array of issues beyond clinical questions. For example, it should have the capacity to address questions about resource allocation, organizational strategy, and community mission. Executives should not only support ethics programs but openly use them in their decision making.

The challenge to leadership is to align the activities of the organization's ethics program or committee with the organization's values and other programs, such as patient safety and quality improvement. The ethics program should be made clear to patients, staff, stakeholders, trustees, and the community served and should be responsive to their needs.

Executives need to support training of members of the organization's ethics program. And ethics program leaders in turn should provide educational offerings to staff, patients, and trustees that are designed to reinforce organizational values, teach ways to resolve situations in which a conflict between observed behaviors and institutional values occurs, and discuss, through the use of actual case studies, how ethical conflicts were brought forward and addressed in the organization.

Effective Ethics Program Checklist

❑ Does leadership openly and publicly support the ethics program?
❑ Are ethics activities integrated into the organization?
❑ Have ethics committee members been trained to address clinical and organization issues?
❑ Do all staff members have access to the ethics program?
❑ Are recurring ethical issues identified and addressed?
❑ Is staff moral distress acknowledged and addressed at every level in the organization?

EXECUTIVE ACTION

The final component in building an ethical culture is having administrative and clinical leaders demonstrate an unwavering commitment to the importance of ethics. Linda Trevino, PhD, of the Pennsylvania State University, noted in a 2005 presentation that executive ethical leadership includes the leader's behavior (moral person)—including traits, personal morality, and values-based decision making—and the leader's ability to direct followers' behavior (moral manager), including role modeling and how the leader rewards and disciplines and communicates the importance of ethics.

Being a model for ethical behaviors is set in day-to-day actions and decisions. Lynn Sharp Paine, in a 1994 *Harvard Business Review* article (vol. 72, no. 2), challenged managers to "acknowledge their role in sharpening organizational ethics and seize this opportunity to create a climate that can strengthen the relationships and reputations on which their companies' success depends." Paine argues the need for organizations to design an ethical framework that is "...no longer a burdensome constraint ... but the governing ethos of the organization."

A key component in role modeling is openly discussing ethics and using the organization's ethics resources. When managerial performance targets are being determined or resource allocation and financial strategy is being decided, are the decisions made within the context of organizational values? When executive leadership establishes and embarks on new capital and strategic projects, such as an expansion of radiation oncology or the construction of a new emergency facility, is the decision reached using an ethically guided decision-making process? Or is it considered simply in the framework of a business decision? The use of an ethically guided decision-making process will assist the organization when making a public announcement about the decision and answering questions that inevitably will be raised about lost opportunities (e.g., not to pursue expansion of home- and community-based services).

It is easy to publicly proclaim how decisions are reached following a process that ensures consistency with values. However, the true test of a leader's adherence to organizational values often comes in the most difficult of times—for example, the leader's willingness to publicly disclose activities such as fraudulent reporting, billing inaccuracies, or safety violations. The Joint Commission requires healthcare organizations to conduct intensive investigations of actual or potential system failures that harm or might have harmed patients. Is leadership willing to take the additional step of widely disclosing the error, the analysis, and the findings?

Ethics Leadership Checklist

❑ Do clinicians' and administrative executives' actions reflect adherence to the organization's values?
❑ Does leadership openly talk about the importance of ethics?

❑ Are executive decision-making processes and decisions transparent?

❑ Do healthcare executives consult with the organization's ethics committee?

❑ Do healthcare executives serve as role models regarding ethical behavior and traits?

An ethics-driven culture is central to quality care. When unethical behaviors or even ethical uncertainty exists, the quality of care can be diminished. Staff members are demoralized and less effective. The organization's culture is a complex dynamic that has evolved over time and includes both formal (policies, staff selection, decision processes, etc.) and informal (rituals, dress, daily employee relations and behavior, language, etc.) systems.

Healthcare executives play a key role in setting the tone for building, maintaining, and, when needed, changing policies so the organization's culture becomes more grounded in ethics. Just as the current culture did not happen by accident or overnight, enhancing the culture will not just happen by chance—it requires attention, thoughtful review, careful planning, and clear leadership. The benefits to an organization of having an ethical culture make the effort worth it.

November/December 2009

PART V:
ACHE ETHICS
RESOURCES

THIS SECTION CONTAINS a wide range of useful documents and tools developed and disseminated by ACHE to help executives maintain their ethical integrity and promote ethical practices within their organizations. Among the nine ACHE Ethical Policy Statements are several updated policies and two new ones— "Considerations for Healthcare Executive–Supplier Interactions" and "Promise-Making, Keeping and Rescinding." In addition, other documents, including the recently revised ACHE *Code of Ethics* and the Ethics Self-Assessment are provided. The section also includes a model for an organizational decision-making process to assist executives and others when addressing ethical challenges.

American College of Healthcare Executives *Code of Ethics**

PREAMBLE

The purpose of the *Code of Ethics* of the American College of Healthcare Executives is to serve as a standard of conduct for affiliates. It contains standards of ethical behavior for healthcare executives in their professional relationships. These relationships include colleagues, patients or others served; members of the healthcare executive's organization and other organizations, the community, and society as a whole.

The *Code of Ethics* also incorporates standards of ethical behavior governing individual behavior, particularly when that conduct directly relates to the role and identity of the healthcare executive.

The fundamental objectives of the healthcare management profession are to maintain or enhance the overall quality of life, dignity and well-being of every individual needing healthcare service and to create a more equitable, accessible, effective and efficient healthcare system.

Healthcare executives have an obligation to act in ways that will merit the trust, confidence, and respect of healthcare professionals and the general public. Therefore, healthcare executives should lead lives that embody an exemplary system of values and ethics.

* As amended by the Board of Governors on March 16, 2007.

In fulfilling their commitments and obligations to patients or others served, healthcare executives function as moral advocates and models. Since every management decision affects the health and well-being of both individuals and communities, healthcare executives must carefully evaluate the possible outcomes of their decisions. In organizations that deliver healthcare services, they must work to safeguard and foster the rights, interests and prerogatives of patients or others served.

The role of moral advocate requires that healthcare executives take actions necessary to promote such rights, interests and prerogatives.

Being a model means that decisions and actions will reflect personal integrity and ethical leadership that others will seek to emulate.

I. THE HEALTHCARE EXECUTIVE'S RESPONSIBILITIES TO THE PROFESSION OF HEALTHCARE MANAGEMENT

The healthcare executive shall:

A. Uphold the *Code of Ethics* and mission of the American College of Healthcare Executives;
B. Conduct professional activities with honesty, integrity, respect, fairness and good faith in a manner that will reflect well upon the profession;
C. Comply with all laws and regulations pertaining to healthcare management in the jurisdictions in which the healthcare executive is located or conducts professional activities;
D. Maintain competence and proficiency in healthcare management by implementing a personal program of assessment and continuing professional education;
E. Avoid the improper exploitation of professional relationships for personal gain;

F. Disclose financial and other conflicts of interest;

G. Use this *Code* to further the interests of the profession and not for selfish reasons;

H. Respect professional confidences;

I. Enhance the dignity and image of the healthcare management profession through positive public information programs; and

J. Refrain from participating in any activity that demeans the credibility and dignity of the healthcare management profession.

II. THE HEALTHCARE EXECUTIVE'S RESPONSIBILITIES TO PATIENTS OR OTHERS SERVED

The healthcare executive shall, within the scope of his or her authority:

A. Work to ensure the existence of a process to evaluate the quality of care or service rendered;

B. Avoid practicing or facilitating discrimination and institute safeguards to prevent discriminatory organizational practices;

C. Work to ensure the existence of a process that will advise patients or others served of the rights, opportunities, responsibilities and risks regarding available healthcare services;

D. Work to ensure that there is a process in place to facilitate the resolution of conflicts that may arise when values of patients and their families differ from those of employees and physicians;

E. Demonstrate zero tolerance for any abuse of power that compromises patients or others served;

F. Work to provide a process that ensures the autonomy and self-determination of patients or others served; and

G. Work to ensure the existence of procedures that will safe-guard the confidentiality and privacy of patients or others served.

III. THE HEALTHCARE EXECUTIVE'S RESPONSIBILITIES TO THE ORGANIZATION

The healthcare executive shall, within the scope of his or her authority:

A. Provide healthcare services consistent with available resources, and when there are limited resources, work to ensure the existence of a resource allocation process that considers ethical ramifications;
B. Conduct both competitive and cooperative activities in ways that improve community healthcare services;
C. Lead the organization in the use and improvement of standards of management and sound business practices;
D. Respect the customs and practices of patients or others served, consistent with the organization's philosophy;
E. Be truthful in all forms of professional and organizational communication, and avoid disseminating information that is false, misleading or deceptive;
F. Report negative financial and other information promptly and accurately, and initiate appropriate action;
G. Prevent fraud and abuse and aggressive accounting practices that may result in disputable financial reports;
H. Create an organizational environment in which both clinical and management mistakes are minimized and, when they do occur, are disclosed and addressed effectively;
I. Implement an organizational code of ethics and monitor compliance; and
J. Provide ethics resources to staff to address organizational and clinical issues.

IV. THE HEALTHCARE EXECUTIVE'S RESPONSIBILITIES TO EMPLOYEES

Healthcare executives have ethical and professional obligations to the employees they manage that encompass but are not limited to:

A. Creating a work environment that promotes ethical conduct by employees;
B. Providing a work environment that encourages a free expression of ethical concerns and provides mechanisms for discussing and addressing such concerns;
C. Providing a work environment that discourages harassment, sexual and other; coercion of any kind, especially to perform illegal or unethical acts; and discrimination on the basis of race, ethnicity, creed, gender, sexual orientation, age, or disability;
D. Providing a work environment that promotes the proper use of employees' knowledge and skills;
E. Providing a safe work environment; and
F. Establishing appropriate grievance and appeals mechanisms.

V. THE HEALTHCARE EXECUTIVE'S RESPONSIBILITIES TO COMMUNITY AND SOCIETY

The healthcare executive shall:

A. Work to identify and meet the healthcare needs of the community;
B. Work to support access to healthcare services for all people;
C. Encourage and participate in public dialogue on healthcare policy issues, and advocate solutions that will improve health status and promote quality healthcare;

D. Apply short- and long-term assessments to management decisions affecting both community and society; and

E. Provide prospective patients and others with adequate and accurate information, enabling them to make enlightened decisions regarding services.

VI. THE HEALTHCARE EXECUTIVE'S RESPONSIBILITY TO REPORT VIOLATIONS OF THE *CODE*

An affiliate of ACHE who has reasonable grounds to believe that another affiliate has violated this *Code* has a duty to communicate such facts to the Ethics Committee.

ADDITIONAL RESOURCES

Available on ache.org or by calling ACHE at (312) 424-2800.

1. ACHE *Ethical Policy Statements*
   - "Considerations for Healthcare Executive-Supplier Interactions"
   - "Creating an Ethical Environment for Employees"
   - "Decisions Near the End of Life"
   - "Ethical Decision Making for Healthcare Executives"
   - "Ethical Issues Related to a Reduction in Force"
   - "Ethical Issues Related to Staff Shortages"
   - "Health Information Confidentiality"
   - "Impaired Healthcare Executives"
   - "Promise-Making, Keeping and Rescinding"
2. ACHE Grievance Procedure
3. ACHE Ethics Committee Action
4. ACHE Ethics Committee Scope and Function

American College of Healthcare Executives
Ethical Policy Statement

Considerations for Healthcare Executive–Supplier Interactions

November 2007

STATEMENT OF THE ISSUE

Healthcare executives share a fundamental commitment to enhance the quality of life and well being of those needing healthcare services and to create a more equitable, effective and efficient healthcare delivery system. To accomplish these fundamental objectives, healthcare executives must rely on an intricate network of professionals that include professionals within the supplier community.

The realm of healthcare executive-supplier relationships involves not only the purchase of goods and services, but also the mutual provision of information and advice.

In interacting with current and potential suppliers, healthcare executives must act in ways that merit trust, confidence and respect, while fulfilling their duties to the public, their organizations and their profession. Further, it is important to avoid even the appearance of conflicts of interest that may seem to unduly advantage the healthcare executive, the organization or the supplier. Thus, healthcare executives must demonstrate the utmost integrity as well as embrace the need for transparency in interactions with suppliers.

POLICY POSITION

The American College of Healthcare Executives believes that healthcare executives should interact with company representatives who sell products and services to their organizations in a way that:

- advances patient care or improves healthcare delivery;
- is fully disclosed to the executive's organization;
- does not damage the reputation of the organization or the profession;
- does not violate applicable law; and
- does not violate policies of the executive's organization.

In determining whether the nature of specific interactions meet each of the above guidelines, healthcare executives should carefully consider the issues detailed below.

1. The interaction between an executive and a supplier can be considered to enhance patient care or improve healthcare delivery when one or more of the following conditions are evident:

    - It furthers the **executive's** knowledge of products or services which may improve patient care.
    - It furthers the **supplier's** knowledge of healthcare needs, so that the supplier can produce better products and services.
    - It facilitates the efficient and cost effective delivery of products and services to the executive's organization.

    Examples of types of interactions that could enhance patient care or improve healthcare delivery are attendance by executives at trade show exhibits of supplier products; seminars or demonstrations produced by suppliers; and participation in supplier advisory councils, supplier surveys, or one-on-one visits with suppliers to exchange ideas.

2. Full disclosure of the supplier-executive relationship to the executive's organization should ordinarily be made to the party within the organization to whom the executive reports (e.g., a supervisor, the CEO or the Board/Chairman) or through the organization's compliance program officer. To prevent misunderstanding, it is advisable that disclosure include all remuneration arrangements, including reimbursements or perquisites (e.g., airfare or meals).

3. Even with full disclosure, damage to the reputation of the executive, the organization or the profession may occur. The executive should avoid interactions with suppliers when this risk is present.
    - Executives should avoid interaction with suppliers that could result in undue influence by suppliers in the decision-making process.
    - As with any position of public trust, avoiding even the appearance of wrongdoing, conflict of interest or interference with free competition is important. Executives should take care that interactions with suppliers not result in perceptions of undue influence or other perceived impropriety.

4. Healthcare executives are subject to the federal anti-kickback statute which makes it a criminal offense to knowingly and willfully offer, pay, solicit or receive any remuneration in order to induce referrals of items or services reimbursable by federal healthcare programs.
    - The anti-kickback statute interprets "remuneration" very broadly, including the transfer of anything of value, in cash or in kind, directly or indirectly, covertly or overtly.
    - The healthcare executive should be aware that other statutes, which may vary from state to state, may also be applicable. If the application of a law is unclear to a

proposed interaction, the executive has a duty to seek guidance from the appropriate party, who may be the person to whom the executive reports or the organization's legal counsel.

5. In addition to applicable laws, healthcare executives have a duty to be familiar and comply with their organizational policies governing interaction with suppliers. If the application of a policy is unclear to a proposed interaction, the executive has a duty to seek guidance from the appropriate party, who may be the person to whom the executive reports, the organization's legal counsel, compliance officer or ethics advisor.

The same type of relationship, such as participating in a supplier produced seminar or a supplier advisory council, may be appropriate, or alternatively, may raise significant questions. The context and nature of the relationship can be more significant than the specific setting or type of interaction. Therefore, in addition to the above criteria, there are a number of questions healthcare executives should consider when assessing the nature of arrangements with suppliers and evaluating if a real or perceived conflict of interest is likely:

*   Will the relationship affect your judgment, the judgment of your colleagues or the organization?
*   Who will benefit from the relationship? Who might suffer?
*   Would you be comfortable with the relationship being known to your patients, stakeholders and the general public?
*   Can you defend the relationship to your colleagues and superiors?
*   Does it represent a positive model for managerial, professional or organizational behavior?
*   Would you expect other organizations or individuals to behave similarly?
*   Is it fair to all parties?

When considering these questions, the healthcare executive should be cognizant of the need for public trust and the avoidance of even the appearance of impropriety. Furthermore, to foster knowledge and sensitivity to potential issues associated with supplier interactions, healthcare executives should promote the dissemination of this policy statement to appropriate managers within their organizations as well as to relevant suppliers.

Approved by the Board of Governors of the American College of Healthcare Executives on November 12, 2007.

American College of Healthcare Executives
Ethical Policy Statement

Creating an Ethical Environment
for Employees

March 1992
August 1995 (revised)
November 2000 (revised)
November 2005 (revised)

STATEMENT OF THE ISSUE

The number and magnitude of challenges facing healthcare organizations are unprecedented. Growing financial pressures, rising
public and payor expectations and the increasing number of consolidations have placed hospitals, health networks, managed care
plans and other healthcare organizations under greater stress—thus
potentially intensifying ethical dilemmas.

Now, more than ever, the healthcare organization must be managed with consistently high professional and ethical standards. This
means that the executive, acting with other responsible parties, must
foster and support an environment conducive not only to providing high-quality, cost-effective healthcare, but also seek to ensure
individual ethical behavior and practices.

Recognizing the importance of ethics, healthcare executives should
seek various ways to integrate ethical practices and reflection into the
organization's overall culture. To create such an ethical environment for
all employees, healthcare executives should: 1.) support the development and implementation of employee ethical standards of behavior

that include ethical clinical and administrative practices, and 2.) ensure effective and competent ethics resources exist and are available to all employees, such as ethics committees to clarify such standards of behavior when there is ethical uncertainty. The executive also must support and implement a systematic and organization-wide approach to ethics training as well as corporate compliance for all staff.

The ability of an organization to achieve its full potential will remain dependent upon the motivation, knowledge, skills and ethical behavior of its staff. Thus, the executive has an obligation to accomplish the organization's mission in a manner that respects the values of individuals and maximizes their contributions.

POLICY POSITION

The American College of Healthcare Executives believes that all healthcare executives have an ethical and professional obligation to employees of the organizations they manage to create a working environment that supports, but is not limited to:

- Reviewing the principles and ideals expressed in vision, mission and value statements, personnel policies, annual reports, employee orientation materials, and other documents to test congruence;
- The development of an organizational code of ethics that includes guidelines for all employees' ethical standards of behavior and practices;
- Responsible employee ethical behavior and practices based on the organization's code of ethics and ethical standards of practice. Such expectations should be included in employee position descriptions where relevant;
- Free expression of ethical concerns;
- An available ethics resource for discussing and addressing clinical, organizational and research related ethical concerns without retribution, such as an ethics committee;

- Establish an anonymous mechanism that safeguards employees who wish to raise ethical concerns;
- Freedom from all harassment, coercion and discrimination;
- Appropriate use of an employee's knowledge, skills and abilities; and
- A safe work environment.

These responsibilities can best be implemented in an environment where all employees are encouraged to develop and adhere to the highest standards of ethics. This should be done with attention to other features of the code of ethics and appropriate professional code, particularly those that stress the moral character of the executive and the organization itself.

Approved by the Board of Governors of the American College of Healthcare Executives on November 7, 2005.

American College of Healthcare Executives Ethical Policy Statement

Decisions Near the End of Life

August 1994
November 1999 (revised)
November 2004 (revised)
November 2009 (revised)

STATEMENT OF THE ISSUE

End-of-life decision making and care are important aspects of the delivery of healthcare. Medical technology has shaped the circumstances of death, giving us options that may impact when, where and how we die. Intervening at the moment of death, technology can now sustain lives even when there is little or no hope for recovery or a meaningful existence. However, such actions may be inconsistent with patient desires and foster unwarranted variations in end-of-life practice patterns.

In response, patients and/or their proxies are exercising more influence over decisions regarding interventions that may prolong existence rather than allowing the natural progression of the dying process near the end of life. The traditional value to preserve life by all possible means is now being weighed against patient-centered, quality-of-life considerations based on evidence-based care and a shared decision-making process.

POLICY POSITION

The American College of Healthcare Executives (ACHE) urges healthcare executives to address the ethical dilemmas and care issues surrounding death and dying. Additionally, executives should promote public dialogue that will lead to awareness and understanding of end-of-life concerns.

ACHE encourages all healthcare executives to play a significant role in addressing this issue by:

Ensuring Ethical End-of-Life Decision Making

- Healthcare executives and their organizations should promote the patient's (or, when lacking decision-making capacity, the authorized surrogate's) self-determination regarding end-of-life decision making. Generally, informed adult patients or their surrogates have the ethical and legal right to accept or refuse any recommended treatments based on the ethical principle of autonomy. Such decision making should include an open, truthful discussion regarding the patient's situation and evidence-driven healthcare options.
- The healthcare executive should ensure that patient or surrogate decisions are appropriately documented and respected.
- When there is disagreement regarding treatments for patients lacking decision-making capacity (even those patients who have valid advance directives or durable power of attorney documents), the guidance of an ethics committee or similar resource may aid in resolution. Healthcare executives should ensure that there are clear guidelines, including a process to address care management disputes as well as provide support to healthcare professionals and families responsible for making treatment choices.

Fostering the Use of Advance Planning Documents

- Healthcare executives should advocate for the introduction, discussion and completion of organ and tissue donation designation and advance directives documents, including a recognized living will and durable power of attorney for healthcare. Ideally, such documents should be prepared prior to hospitalization or a medical crisis (see related *Policy Statement,* "Organ/Tissue/Blood/Blood Stem Cells Donation Process").

- When the patient lacks decision-making capacity, treatment decisions should conform to what the patient would want based on his or her written or oral advance directive. In the absence of clear advance directives, the designated surrogate should be the decision maker and act in accordance with his or her understanding of the patient's desires.

Developing and Implementing End-of-Life Organizational Guidelines

- Healthcare executives should ensure that appropriate end-of-life care and decision-making policies and procedures are developed and implemented, including do-not-resuscitate orders, withholding and withdrawing life-sustaining treatment, medical futility, and organ donation. Such guidelines should be regularly reviewed.
- When developing and implementing guidelines, healthcare executives should encourage cooperation and understanding among the clinical staff, members of the governing body, and executive management. Executives should ensure that appropriate methods for raising awareness and staff education are provided regarding end-of-life ethical dilemmas, including how to access organizational ethics resources.
- If organizational policies limit specific end-of-life options for patients and families or surrogates, healthcare executives have a responsibility to see that procedures are in place that provide disclosure of such limitations.

Ensuring Available End-of-Life Care Support for Patients, Families and Staff Members

- In the care of patients at the end of life, executives should support the development and availability of effective resources such as palliative care and hospice programs for patients and families to preserve psychological, social, and spiritual well-being.
- Executives should support the development of resources and programs that promote pain control as a crucial modality in the management of patients at the end of life.
- Executives should ensure that staff have the knowledge and resources to address end-of-life decision making and patient care.
- Executives should ensure that effective support programs, such as ethics committees and employee assistance, are available to staff members to address ethical conflicts and moral distress that frequently surround end-of-life decision making and patient care.

Promoting Community End-of-Life Discussion

- Executives should heighten awareness of ethical issues, including the patient or surrogate's right to choose treatment, through information forums that promote open discussion among patients and their families, attorneys, clergy members, journalists, physicians, and other healthcare professionals. By raising and openly discussing ethics issues, healthcare executives will aid the public in understanding the importance of thinking about end-of-life issues and the organization's interest in ensuring patient-centered care.

Healthcare executives should foster reasoned, compassionate, patient-centered decision making that considers the rights and values of patients and staff members. While interpretation of these principles will vary by local custom and law, healthcare executives have a responsibility to ensure their organization operates with respect for the inherent worth and human dignity of every individual.

Related Resource

American College of Healthcare Executives *Policy Statement*, "Organ/Tissue/Blood/Blood Stem Cells Donation Process."

Approved by the Board of Governors of the American College of Healthcare Executives on November 16, 2009.

American College of Healthcare Executives
Ethical Policy Statement

Ethical Decision Making for Healthcare Executives

August 1993
February 1997 (revised)
November 2002 (revised)
November 2007 (revised)

STATEMENT OF THE ISSUE

Ethical decision making is required when the healthcare executive must balance the needs and interests of the individual, the organization and society. Those involved in this decision making process must consider ethical principles such as justice, autonomy, beneficence and fairness, as well as professional ethical standards and codes. Many factors have contributed to the growing concern in healthcare organizations with ethical issues, including issues of access and affordability, pressure to reduce costs, mergers and acquisitions, financial and other resource constraints, and advances in medical technology that complicate decision making near the end of life. Healthcare executives have a responsibility to address the growing number of complex ethical dilemmas they are facing, but they cannot and should not make such decisions alone or without a sound decision-making framework.

Healthcare organizations should have vehicles that may include ethics committees, ethics consultation services, processes for dealing with potential conflicts of interest or written policies and procedures to assist healthcare executives with the ethics decision-making process. With these organizational mechanisms, the sometimes conflicting interests of patients, families, caregivers, the organization, payors, and the community can be appropriately weighed and balanced.

POLICY POSITION

It is incumbent upon healthcare executives to lead in a manner that sets an ethical tone for their organizations. The American College of Healthcare Executives (ACHE) believes education in ethics is an important step in a healthcare executive's lifelong commitment to high ethical conduct, both personally and professionally. Further, ACHE supports the development of organizational mechanisms that enable healthcare executives to appropriately and expeditiously address ethical dilemmas. Whereas physicians, nurses and other caregivers may primarily address ethical issues on a case-by-case basis, healthcare executives also have a responsibility to address those issues at broader organizational, community and societal levels. ACHE encourages its affiliates, as leaders in their organizations, to take an active role in the development and demonstration of ethical decision making.

To this end, healthcare executives should:

- Seek to create a culture that fosters ethical practices and ethical decision making throughout the organization.
- Communicate the organization's commitment to ethical decision making through its mission or value statements and its organizational code of ethics.
- Demonstrate through their professional behavior the importance of ethics to the organization.
- Offer educational programs to boards, staff, physicians and others on their organization's ethical standards of practice and on the more global issues of ethical decision making in today's healthcare environment. Further, healthcare executives should

promote learning opportunities, such as those provided through professional societies or academic organizations, that will facilitate open discussion of ethical issues.

- Develop and use organizational mechanisms that reflect their organizations' mission and values and are flexible enough to deal with the spectrum of ethical concerns—clinical, organizational, business and management.
- Ensure that organizational mechanisms to address ethics issues are readily available, and include individuals who are competent to address ethical concerns and reflect diverse perspectives. An organization's ethics committee, for example, might include representatives from groups such as physicians, nurses, managers, board members, social workers, attorneys, patient and/or community representatives, and clergy. All these groups are likely to bring unique and valuable perspectives to bear on discussions of ethical issues.
- Evaluate and continually refine organizational processes for addressing ethical issues.
- Promote decision making that results in the appropriate use of power while balancing individual, organizational and societal issues.

Approved by the Board of Governors of the American College of Healthcare Executives on November 12, 2007.

American College of Healthcare Executives Ethical Policy Statement

Ethical Issues Related to a Reduction in Force

August 1995
November 2000 (revised)
November 2005 (revised)

STATEMENT OF THE ISSUE

As the result of managed care, such as variable admissions, shorter lengths of stay, higher productivity, new technology, and other factors, the capacity of some healthcare organizations could significantly exceed demand. As a result, these organizations may be required to reduce their work force. Additionally, mergers and consolidations can result in further reductions and reassignments of staff. Financial pressures will continue to fuel this trend. However, patient care needs should not be compromised when determining staffing requirements.

Careful planning, diligent cost controls, effective resource management, and proper consultation can lessen the hardship and stress of a reduction in force. Formal policies and procedures should be developed well in advance of the need to implement them.

The decision to reduce staff necessitates consideration of the short-term and long-term impact on all employees—those leaving and those remaining. Decision makers should consider the potential ethical conflict between formally stated organizational values and staff reduction actions.

POLICY POSITION

The American College of Healthcare Executives recommends that specific steps be considered by healthcare executives when initiating a reduction in force process to support consistency between stated organizational values and those demonstrated before, during and after the process. Among these steps are the following:

- Recognize that cost reduction efforts must be appropriate—if they are too aggressive, the consequences for patients, staff and the organization can be as harmful as doing too little or proceeding too late;
- Consult with labor counsel;
- Provide timely, accurate, clear and consistent information—including the reasoning behind the decision—to stakeholders when staff reductions become necessary;
- Review the principles and ideals expressed in vision, mission and value statements, personnel policies, annual reports, employee orientation materials, and other documents to test congruence and conformance with reduction in force decisions;
- Support, if possible, through retraining and redeployment, employees whose positions have been eliminated. Also, consider outplacement assistance and appropriate severance policies, if possible; and
- Address the needs of remaining staff by demonstrating sensitivity to their potential feelings of loss, anger and survivor guilt. Also address their anxiety about the possibility of further reductions, uncertainty regarding changes in workload, work redesign, and similar concerns.

Healthcare organizations encounter the same set of challenging issues associated with reductions in force as do other employers. Reduction in force decisions should reflect an institution's ethics and value statements.

Approved by the Board of Governors of the American College of Healthcare Executives on November 7, 2005.

American College of Healthcare Executives Ethical Policy Statement

Ethical Issues Related to Staff Shortages

March 2002
November 2007 (revised)

STATEMENT OF THE ISSUE

The effects of staff shortages are felt acutely by hospitals and other healthcare organizations. While less than a decade ago healthcare executives were struggling with how to reduce their organization's staff responsibly, today they face an equally daunting challenge. They must fulfill their responsibility to provide high-quality, affordable patient care in the face of work force shortages that may leave them with vacancies in many positions throughout their organization.

Alleviating work force shortages or adapting to them is a complex problem for which there are few easy solutions. Nevertheless, healthcare executives have an ethical responsibility to address any shortages that exist within their organizations in such a way that patient care is not compromised, existing staff are not unduly burdened and financial costs do not become excessive.

POLICY POSITION

The American College of Healthcare Executives (ACHE) recommends that healthcare executives develop responsible action plans for delivering patient care in the face of staff shortages. To this end, ACHE recommends that such plans address the following:

- Attracting and retaining qualified staff by addressing issues important to today's work force, including strengthening the patient/clinician/executive partnership, treating each other with respect, promoting continuous quality improvement, and providing fair compensation, flexible scheduling and professional development;
- Maintaining workloads and expectations that strive to alleviate and prevent burnout;
- Creating systems for job assignments and backup coverage that ensure responsibilities are appropriately matched with qualifications;
- Being sensitive to the financial and nonfinancial consequences of utilizing temporary personnel to fill vacancies;
- Responding to potential disasters that would significantly impact staff availability over sustained periods, requiring multilevel backup capacity;
- Conducting employee opinion surveys and exit interviews, using results to identify steps to improve job satisfaction;
- Identifying ways to engage employees to help define and address issues adversely affecting recruitment and retention objectives;
- Maintaining a diverse and culturally competent work force;
- Analyzing departments or units with high turnover rates to determine whether management shortcomings, working conditions, and/or other factors may be contributing to staff morale problems; and
- Closing units or diverting patients if staff shortages become severe, to ensure that patient care is not compromised and high-quality care is maintained.

Healthcare executives may find it beneficial to join forces with others in their service areas to address the problem of staff shortages.

Collaboration to recruit qualified staff will prove to be a more effective long-term strategy than competition for the same resources. ACHE encourages healthcare executives to collaborate on the development of creative, sustainable strategies that will benefit their respective organizations as well as help ensure that high-quality, affordable healthcare remains available in their communities.

In addition, ACHE encourages healthcare executives to work to ensure the future supply of healthcare workers. Healthcare executives should collaborate with others to expose students to careers in healthcare, including both clinical and managerial careers.

Approved by the Board of Governors of the American College of Healthcare Executives on November 12, 2007.

American College of Healthcare Executives
Ethical Policy Statement

Health Information Confidentiality

February 1994
November 1997 (revised)
November 2004 (revised)
November 2009 (revised)

STATEMENT OF THE ISSUE

Healthcare is among the most personal services rendered in our society; yet to deliver this care, scores of personnel must have access to intimate patient information. In order to receive appropriate care, patients must feel free to reveal personal information. In return, the healthcare provider must treat patient information confidentially and protect its security.

Maintaining confidentiality is becoming more difficult. While information technology can improve the quality of care through the instant retrieval and exchange of medical information by a greater number of people who can contribute to the care and treatment of a patient, it also can increase the risk of unauthorized use, access and disclosure of confidential patient information. Within healthcare organizations, personal information contained in medical records now is reviewed not only by physicians and nurses but also by professionals in many clinical and administrative support areas.

The need to protect patient confidentiality is evident in legal restrictions imposed by state laws and the federal Health Insurance Portability and Accountability Act of 1996 (HIPAA) and as recently amended under the Health Information Technology for Economic and Clinical Health Act (the "HITECH Act"). Health information cannot be used or disclosed without proper authorization by patients or legal representatives except under very limited circumstances, such as to promote public health, protect children and spouses from abuse, or otherwise comply with certain laws.

While media representatives also seek access to health information, particularly when a patient is a public figure or when treatment involves legal or public health issues, the rights of individual patients must be protected. Society's need for information rarely outweighs the right of patients to confidentiality.

In order to release patient information, healthcare executives must determine that patients or their legal representatives have consented to the release of information or that the use, access, or disclosure sought falls within the exceptions that do not require the patient's prior consent. Once health information is released, healthcare executives must keep records of most disclosures for review upon patient request.

POLICY POSITION

The American College of Healthcare Executives believes that in addition to following all applicable state laws and HIPAA, healthcare executives have a moral and professional obligation to respect confidentiality and protect the security of patients' medical records. As patient advocates, executives must ensure their organization obtains proper patient authorization to release information or follow carefully defined policies and applicable laws in those cases for which the release of information without consent is indicated.

While the healthcare organization possesses the health record, outside access to the information in that record can be controlled by patients unless indicated otherwise by applicable laws and regulations. Organizations therefore must determine the appropriateness of all requests for patient information under applicable federal and state law and act accordingly.

In fulfilling their responsibilities, healthcare executives should seek to:

- Limit access to patient information to authorized individuals only.
- Ensure that institutional policies on confidentiality, security, and release of information are consistent with regulations and laws.
- Educate healthcare personnel on confidentiality and data security requirements, take steps to ensure all healthcare personnel are aware of and understand their responsibilities to keep patient information confidential and secure, and impose sanctions for violations.
- Safeguard medical record files and computerized data with security and storage systems (including, if appropriate, the use of encryption) that protect against unauthorized use, access, and disclosure and ensure data integrity and availability.
- Develop systems that enable organizations to track (and, if required, report) the use, access, and disclosure of health records.
- Provide for appropriate disaster recovery.
- Establish guidelines for masking patient identifiers in committee minutes and other working documents in which the identity is not necessary.
- Establish policies and procedures to provide to the patient an accounting of uses and disclosures of the patient's health information.
- Create guidelines for securing necessary permissions for the release of medical information for research, education, utilization review, and other purposes.
- Adopt a specialized process to further protect sensitive information such as psychiatric records, HIV status, genetic testing information, sexually transmitted disease information, or substance abuse treatment records.
- Identify special situations that require consultation with senior management prior to use or release of information.
- Obtain written agreements that detail the obligations of confidentiality and security for individuals, third parties and agencies that receive medical records information, unless the circumstances warrant an exception.

- Conduct due diligence on third parties who will receive medical records information, including a review of policies and procedures appropriate to the type of information they will possess. Ensure where applicable that such third parties adhere to the same terms and restrictions regarding protected health information applicable to the organization.
- Follow all applicable policies and procedures regarding privacy of patient information even if information is in the public domain.
- Adopt procedures to address patient rights to request amendment of medical records and other rights under the HIPAA Privacy Rule.
- Educate patients about organizational policies on confidentiality and use the notice of privacy practices as required by the HIPAA Privacy Rule.
- Establish adequate policies and procedures to ensure notification of the affected patient or organization without unreasonable delay, in the event of an occurrence of unauthorized use, access, or disclosure of health information or of a security breach incident.
- In the event of a security breach, conduct a timely and thorough investigation and notify patients promptly if appropriate to mitigate harm in accordance with applicable state or federal law.
- Establish adequate policies and procedures to mitigate the harm caused by the unauthorized use, access, or disclosure of health information to the extent required by state or federal law.
- Participate in the public dialogue on confidentiality issues such as employer use of healthcare information, public health reporting, and appropriate uses and disclosures of information in health information exchanges.

The American College of Healthcare Executives urges all healthcare executives to maintain an appropriate balance between the patient's right to confidentiality and the need to release information in the public's interest in accordance with applicable state and federal law.

Approved by the Board of Governors of the American College of Healthcare Executives on November 16, 2009.

American College of Healthcare Executives Ethical Policy Statement

Impaired Healthcare Executives

February 1991
March 1995 (revised)
November 2000 (revised)
November 2005 (revised)
November 2006 (revised)

STATEMENT OF THE ISSUE

The American College of Healthcare Executives recognizes that impairment, defined broadly to include alcoholism, substance abuse, chemical dependency, mental/emotional instability or cognitive impairment, is a significant problem that crosses all societal boundaries.

Impairment occurs when the healthcare executive is unable to perform professional duties as expected. Impaired healthcare executives affect not only themselves and their families, but they also have a significant impact on their profession; their professional society; their organizations, colleagues, patients, clients and others served; their communities; and society as a whole. Impairment typically leads to misconduct in the form of incompetence and unsafe or unprofessional behavior, which also can lead to substantial costs associated with loss of productivity and errors in judgment.

The impaired healthcare executive can damage the public image of his or her organization of employment. Public confidence in the organization diminishes if it appears that the organization is not being managed with consistently high standards of professional and ethical practice. This lack of public confidence may cause the community to deem the organization unworthy of its support.

Society expects healthcare executives to practice the standards of good health that they advocate for the public. Impaired healthcare executives diminish the credibility of the profession and its ability to manage society's healthcare when they are not appropriately managing their own personal health.

POLICY POSITION

The preamble of the American College of Healthcare Executives *Code of Ethics* states, "Healthcare executives have an obligation to act in ways that will merit the trust, confidence and respect of healthcare professionals and the general public. To do this, healthcare executives must lead lives that embody an exemplary system of values and ethics."

The American College of Healthcare Executives believes that all healthcare executives have an ethical and a professional obligation to:

- Maintain a personal health that is free from impairment.
- Refrain from all professional activities if impaired.
- Expeditiously seek treatment if impairment occurs.
- Urge impaired colleagues to expeditiously seek treatment and to refrain from all professional activities while impaired.
- Assist recovered colleagues when they resume their professional activities.
- Intervene and report the impairment to the appropriate person(s) should the colleague refuse to seek professional assistance and should the state of impairment persist.
- Support peers who identify healthcare executives in need of help.
- Recognize that individuals who have successfully received treatment for impairment and are no longer deemed impaired should be considered for employment opportunities for which they are qualified.

- Recommend or provide, within one's employing organization, confidential avenues for reporting impairment and either access or referral to treatment or assistance programs.
- Urge the community to provide information and resources for assistance and treatment of alcoholism, substance abuse, mental/emotional instability and cognitive impairment as needed and as appropriate.
- Raise the awareness of key stakeholders (such as employees, governing board members, etc.) on impairment issues and the resources available for assistance.

Approved by the Board of Governors of the American College of Healthcare Executives on November 6, 2006.

American College of Healthcare Executives
Ethical Policy Statement

Promise-Making,
Keeping, and Rescinding

March 2006

STATEMENT OF THE ISSUE

In today's environment, healthcare executives are faced with making challenging and complex decisions that require balancing the current and future needs of the overall organization with various constituencies that serve and are served by the organization. Sometimes these decisions come about when healthcare executives are faced with making "promises" or revisiting previous promises made by executives. When this happens, new challenges can come about from the difficult task of weighing the needs of varied constituencies and the use of resources, not to mention the ethical responsibility to make such decisions.

Promises are verbal or written commitments made to another person or group of people. Promises can be formal written agreements, such as contracts, or informal agreements such as when a healthcare executive states to someone (or a group of people) an intention to do something. When the executive does the latter and recognizes that such a statement of intention will lead the person(s) to whom it is given to count on your following through, your statement of intention is a promise. Once made, adhering to a promise is a moral responsibility of the healthcare executive, even if made by one's predecessor.

Despite the moral responsibility that one ought to respect a promise, organizational circumstances may change sufficiently so that the promise should be reviewed, even though the promise may have become a long-standing tradition or expectation. This could be a situation regardless of whether the promise was made by the current healthcare executive or a prior executive in the same position.

However, because trust and honoring moral commitments are hallmarks of successful healthcare organizations, making, revising or rescinding a promise requires thoughtful consideration. A healthcare executive needs sufficient reasons for both making a promise and for breaking a promise. In the latter case, the violation or breaking of a promise without adequate reason leads to harm, not only to the person(s) to whom the promise was made, but also to the executive and the image of the healthcare organization.

POLICY POSITION

Making a Promise

The American College of Healthcare Executives (ACHE) firmly believes that healthcare executives have an ethical responsibility to use a systematic, deliberative and thoughtful approach to decision making when making a promise to a person or a group of people. To ensure such an approach, the following questions should be considered:

- What are the circumstances surrounding the promise? Why is the promise being considered? Why now?
- What are the facts regarding the promise? Is the promise legally binding? What does legal counsel suggest?

- What are the relevant ethical considerations regarding the promise? Is there an ethical rationale for justifying the promise?
- What are the options, such as maintaining the promise, rescinding the promise or altering the promise? Will future CEOs be able to uphold this promise? Are there circumstances under which this promise can or should be revisited? If so, what are they?
- What are the implications (benefits and harms) surrounding the above option(s)? How certain are you of those implications?
- What are the perspectives of the stakeholders affected by the promise?
- Have you carefully reflected on the various options, including conducting a quantitative and qualitative analysis of each option and assessing both the short- and long-term ramifications of each option?
- After selecting a particular option, did you seek the appropriate approval, such as the board's?
- How is the promise going to be communicated and documented? Has this document been shared with the relevant stakeholders? Is it clear how future CEOs will know this promise exists?

Keeping or Rescinding a Promise

1. Making a Decision Regarding a Previous Promise

   After clearly identifying and acknowledging the need to review whether a promise ought to be maintained, the following questions should be considered:

   - What are the circumstances surrounding the promise? Why was the promise made? Why is it being questioned now?
   - What are the facts regarding the promise? Is the promise legally obligated? What does legal counsel suggest?

- What are the relevant ethical considerations regarding maintaining, revising or rescinding the promise? Is there an ethical rationale for justifying the rescinding or revising of the promise?
- What are the options, such as maintaining the promise, rescinding the promise or altering the promise?
- What are the implications (benefits and harms) surrounding each option? How certain are you of those implications?
- What are the perspectives of the stakeholders affected by the promise?
- Have you carefully reflected on the various options, including conducting a quantitative and qualitative analysis of each option and assessing both the short- and long-term ramifications of each option?
- After selecting a particular option, did you seek the appropriate approval, such as the board's, giving the ethical grounding for the decision?

2. Implementing a Decision Regarding a Previous Promise

Decisions to rescind or revise an existing promise should be communicated in a timely manner to all key stakeholders, including the rationale for the action. When decisions are made to revise or rescind a promise, a clear communication plan is advised.

A comprehensive communication plan includes the following:

- Identifying the key audiences and messages.
- Choosing the appropriate spokesperson for the target audience.
- Obtaining the affected stakeholder perspectives and feedback, including being prepared to justify the decision and respond to all questions of concern.

- Considering the response if the decision was reported by the media.
- During the communication process, if concerns or ramifications concerning the action arise that were not previously considered, executives should consider whether to review their decision regarding the promise.

Whether making a promise or reviewing a previous promise, the best decision outcome will be achieved when thoughtful, systematic reasoning and transparency serve as the primary guides for executive behavior.

Common Morality: Deciding What to Do. Bernard Gert. Oxford: University Press 2004. (This is a general reference specifically related to the definition paragraph)

Approved by the Board of Governors of the American College of Healthcare Executives on March 24, 2006.

Ethics Self-Assessment

PURPOSE OF THE ETHICS SELF-ASSESSMENT

Affiliates of the American College of Healthcare Executives agree, as a condition of membership, to abide by ACHE's *Code of Ethics*. The *Code* provides an overall standard of conduct and includes specific standards of ethical behavior to guide healthcare executives in their professional relationships.

Based on the *Code of Ethics*, the Ethics Self-Assessment is intended for your personal use to assist you in thinking about your ethics-related leadership and actions. *It should not be returned to ACHE nor should it be used as a tool for evaluating the ethical behavior of others.*

The Ethics Self-Assessment can help you identify those areas in which you are on strong ethical ground; areas that you may wish to examine the basis for your responses; and opportunities for further reflection. The Ethics Self-Assessment does not have a scoring mechanism, as we do not believe that ethical behavior can or should be quantified.

HOW TO USE THIS SELF-ASSESSMENT

We hope you find this self-assessment thought-provoking and useful as a part of your reflection on applying the ACHE *Code of Ethics* to your everyday activities. You are to be commended for taking time out of your busy schedule to complete it.

Once you have finished the self-assessment, it is suggested that you review your responses, noting which questions you answered "usually," "occasionally" and "almost never." You may find that in some cases an answer of "usually" is satisfactory, but in other cases such as when answering a question about protecting staff's well-being, an answer of "usually" may raise an ethical red flag.

We are confident that you will uncover few red flags where your responses are not compatible with the ACHE *Code of Ethics*. For those you may discover, you should use it as an opportunity to enhance your ethical practice and leadership by developing a specific action plan. For example, you may have noted in the self-assessment that you have not used your organization's ethics mechanism to assist you in addressing challenging ethical conflicts. As a result of this insight you might meet with the chair of the ethics committee to better understand the committee's functions, including case consultation activities, and how you might access this resource when future ethical conflicts arise.

We also want you to consider ACHE as a resource when you and your management team are confronted with difficult ethical dilemmas. In the About ACHE area of **ache.org**, you can access an Ethics Toolkit, a group of practical resources that will help you understand how to integrate ethics into your organization. In addition, you can refer to our regular "Healthcare Management Ethics" column in *Healthcare Executive* magazine, and you may want to consider attending our annual ethics seminar.

Please check one answer for each of the following questions.

I. Leadership

I take courageous, consistent and appropriate management actions to overcome barriers to achieving my organization's mission.

Almost Never   Occasionally   Usually   Always   Not Applicable

I place community/patient benefit over my personal gain.

Almost Never   Occasionally   Usually   Always   Not Applicable

I strive to be a role model for ethical behavior.

Almost Never   Occasionally   Usually   Always   Not Applicable

I work to ensure that decisions about access to care are based primarily on medical necessity, not only on the ability to pay.

Almost Never   Occasionally   Usually   Always   Not Applicable

My statements and actions are consistent with professional ethical standards, including the ACHE *Code of Ethics*.

Almost Never   Occasionally   Usually   Always   Not Applicable

My statements and actions are honest even when circumstances would allow me to confuse the issues.

Almost Never   Occasionally   Usually   Always   Not Applicable

I advocate ethical decision making by the board, management team and medical staff.

Almost Never   Occasionally   Usually   Always   Not Applicable

I use an ethical approach to conflict resolution.

Almost Never   Occasionally   Usually   Always   Not Applicable

I initiate and encourage discussion of the ethical aspects of management/financial issues.

Almost Never   Occasionally   Usually   Always   Not Applicable

I initiate and promote discussion of controversial issues affecting community/patient health (e.g., domestic and community violence and decisions near the end of life).

Almost Never   Occasionally   Usually   Always   Not Applicable

I promptly and candidly explain to internal and external stakeholders negative economic trends and encourage appropriate action.

Almost Never   Occasionally   Usually   Always   Not Applicable

I use my authority solely to fulfill my responsibilities and not for self-interest or to further the interests of family, friends or associates.

Almost Never   Occasionally   Usually   Always   Not Applicable

When an ethical conflict confronts my organization or me, I am successful in finding an effective resolution process and ensure it is followed.

Almost Never   Occasionally   Usually   Always   Not Applicable

I demonstrate respect for my colleagues, superiors and staff.

Almost Never   Occasionally   Usually   Always   Not Applicable

I demonstrate my organization's vision, mission and value statements in my actions.

Almost Never   Occasionally   Usually   Always   Not Applicable

I make timely decisions rather than delaying them to avoid difficult or politically risky choices.

Almost Never   Occasionally   Usually   Always   Not Applicable

I seek the advice of the ethics committee when making ethically challenging decisions.

Almost Never   Occasionally   Usually   Always   Not Applicable

My personal expense reports are accurate and are only billed to a single organization.

Almost Never   Occasionally   Usually   Always   Not Applicable

I openly support establishing and monitoring internal mechanisms (e.g., an ethics committee or program) to support ethical decision making.

Almost Never   Occasionally   Usually   Always   Not Applicable

I thoughtfully consider decisions when making a promise on behalf of the organization to a person or a group of people.

Almost Never   Occasionally   Usually   Always   Not Applicable

II. Relationships

Community

I promote community health status improvement as a guiding goal of my organization and as a cornerstone of my efforts on behalf of my organization.

Almost Never   Occasionally   Usually   Always   Not Applicable

I personally devote time to developing solutions to community health problems.

Almost Never   Occasionally   Usually   Always   Not Applicable

I participate in and encourage my management team to devote personal time to community service.

Almost Never   Occasionally   Usually   Always   Not Applicable

Patients and Their Families

I use a patient- and family-centered approach to patient care.

Almost Never   Occasionally   Usually   Always   Not Applicable

I am a patient advocate on both clinical and financial matters.

Almost Never   Occasionally   Usually   Always   Not Applicable

I ensure equitable treatment of patients regardless of their socioeconomic status, ethnicity or payor category.

Almost Never   Occasionally   Usually   Always   Not Applicable

I respect the practices and customs of a diverse patient population while maintaining the organization's mission.

Almost Never   Occasionally   Usually   Always   Not Applicable

I demonstrate through organizational policies and personal actions that overtreatment and undertreatment of patients are unacceptable.

Almost Never Occasionally Usually Always Not Applicable

I protect patients' rights to autonomy through access to full, accurate information about their illnesses, treatment options and related costs and benefits.

Almost Never Occasionally Usually Always Not Applicable

I promote a patient's right to privacy, including medical record confidentiality, and do not tolerate breaches of this confidentiality.

Almost Never Occasionally Usually Always Not Applicable

Board

I have a routine system in place for board members to make full disclosure and reveal potential conflicts of interest.

Almost Never Occasionally Usually Always Not Applicable

I ensure that reports to the board, my own or others', appropriately convey risks of decisions or proposed projects.

Almost Never Occasionally Usually Always Not Applicable

I work to keep the board focused on ethical issues of importance to the organization, community and other stakeholders.

Almost Never Occasionally Usually Always Not Applicable

I keep the board appropriately informed of patient safety and quality indicators.

Almost Never Occasionally Usually Always Not Applicable

I promote board discussion of resource allocation issues, particularly those where organizational and community interests may appear to be incompatible.

Almost Never Occasionally Usually Always Not Applicable

I keep the board appropriately informed about issues of alleged financial malfeasance, clinical malpractice and potential litigious situations involving employees.

Almost Never Occasionally Usually Always Not Applicable

Colleagues and Staff

I foster discussions about ethical concerns when they arise.

    Almost Never   Occasionally   Usually   Always   Not Applicable

I maintain confidences entrusted to me.

    Almost Never   Occasionally   Usually   Always   Not Applicable

I demonstrate through personal actions and organizational policies zero tolerance for any form of staff harassment.

    Almost Never   Occasionally   Usually   Always   Not Applicable

I encourage discussions about and advocate for the implementation of the organization's code of ethics and value statements.

    Almost Never   Occasionally   Usually   Always   Not Applicable

I fulfill the promises I make.

    Almost Never   Occasionally   Usually   Always   Not Applicable

I am respectful of views different from mine.

    Almost Never   Occasionally   Usually   Always   Not Applicable

I am respectful of individuals who differ from me in ethnicity, gender, education or job position.

    Almost Never   Occasionally   Usually   Always   Not Applicable

I convey negative news promptly and openly, not allowing employees or others to be misled.

    Almost Never   Occasionally   Usually   Always   Not Applicable

I expect and hold staff accountable for adherence to our organization's ethical standards (e.g., performance reviews).

    Almost Never   Occasionally   Usually   Always   Not Applicable

I demonstrate that incompetent supervision is not tolerated and make timely decisions regarding marginally performing managers.

Almost Never   Occasionally   Usually   Always   Not Applicable

I ensure adherence to ethics-related policies and practices affecting patients and staff.

Almost Never   Occasionally   Usually   Always   Not Applicable

I am sensitive to employees who have ethical concerns and facilitate resolution of these concerns.

Almost Never   Occasionally   Usually   Always   Not Applicable

I encourage the use of organizational mechanisms (e.g., an ethics committee or program) and other ethics resources to address ethical issues.

Almost Never   Occasionally   Usually   Always   Not Applicable

I act quickly and decisively when employees are not treated fairly in their relationships with other employees.

Almost Never   Occasionally   Usually   Always   Not Applicable

I assign staff only to official duties and do not ask them to assist me with work on behalf of my family, friends or associates.

Almost Never   Occasionally   Usually   Always   Not Applicable

I hold all staff and clinical/business partners accountable for compliance with professional standards, including ethical behavior.

Almost Never   Occasionally   Usually   Always   Not Applicable

Clinicians

When problems arise with clinical care, I ensure that the problems receive prompt attention and resolution by the responsible parties.

Almost Never   Occasionally   Usually   Always   Not Applicable

I insist that my organization's clinical practice guidelines are consistent with our vision, mission, value statements and ethical standards of practice.

Almost Never   Occasionally   Usually   Always   Not Applicable

When practice variations in care suggest quality of care is at stake, I encourage timely actions that serve patients' interests.

Almost Never   Occasionally   Usually   Always   Not Applicable

I insist that participating clinicians and staff live up to the terms of managed care contracts.

Almost Never   Occasionally   Usually   Always   Not Applicable

I encourage clinicians to access ethics resources when ethical conflicts occur.

Almost Never   Occasionally   Usually   Always   Not Applicable

I encourage resource allocation that is equitable, is based on clinical needs and appropriately balances patient needs and organizational/clinical resources.

Almost Never   Occasionally   Usually   Always   Not Applicable

I expeditiously and forthrightly deal with impaired clinicians and take necessary action when I believe a clinician is not competent to perform his/her clinical duties.

Almost Never   Occasionally   Usually   Always   Not Applicable

I expect and hold clinicians accountable for adhering to their professional and the organization's ethical practices.

Almost Never   Occasionally   Usually   Always   Not Applicable

Buyers, Payers, and Suppliers

I negotiate and expect my management team to negotiate in good faith.

Almost Never   Occasionally   Usually   Always   Not Applicable

I am mindful of the importance of avoiding even the appearance of wrongdoing, conflict of interest, or interference with free competition.

Almost Never   Occasionally   Usually   Always   Not Applicable

I personally disclose and expect board members, staff members and clinicians to disclose any possible conflicts of interests before pursuing or entering into relationships with potential business partners.

Almost Never   Occasionally   Usually   Always   Not Applicable

I promote familiarity and compliance with organizational policies governing relationships with buyers, payors and suppliers.

Almost Never   Occasionally   Usually   Always   Not Applicable

I set an example for others in my organization by not accepting personal gifts from suppliers.

Almost Never   Occasionally   Usually   Always   Not Applicable

An Organizational Ethics Decision-Making Process

William A. Nelson, PhD

THE MANAGEMENT TEAM of Memorial Medical Center must make a decision regarding the continuation of one of its outpatient clinics. To provide better community service, MMC developed three outpatient clinics throughout a large metropolitan area. Over the past several years, one of the clinics has consistently been a financial loser. The losses have grown even as the costs of maintaining the clinic have increased. A primary reason for the negative financial performance is the high amount of nonreimbursed healthcare services—the clinic provides needed healthcare to a low-income part of the metropolitan area. Several members of the executive management team believe MMC has no alternative other than closing the clinic. One member of the management team, however, believes that the situation raises ethical concerns, and that executive seeks an ethics-grounded response to the problem.

For many healthcare executives, ethical conflicts like the one described above are regular occurrences. The nature of healthcare management is such that decisions with ethical implications are made every day—for issues as diverse as access to the organization's services, a particular employee's behavior, clinical practices, and the allocation of limited resources. The decisions made and actions taken in response to ethical questions are critical because of their direct impact on the quality of care. Does your organization have an effective ethics infrastructure in place that includes a structured process to address ethical conflicts?

THE CONCEPT OF PROCEDURAL JUSTICE

At the foundation of organizational ethical decision making is the application of the concept of procedural justice—organizations should rely on a deliberative process to foster fairness through a clear understanding of all competing values in response to a particular ethical conflict. The belief is that if the process is fair, the outcome will more likely be fair as well. To do this, decision makers must take into account the perceptions and values of those affected by the decision and explore various options and how the options are driven by underlying values. Once the options and their underlying values are understood, decision makers choose from the value-driven options. The result of the decision-making process should be openly shared, including the reasoning driving the decision, and there should be a feedback loop for reviewing the outcome of the decision. Such a process is not an algorithm providing one clear answer to every ethical conflict but rather a method to understand different perspectives to the problem, organize and prioritize one's thinking, and appreciate the implications of various options.

The procedural justice approach, similar to the stakeholder theory in business ethics, takes into account the rights, values, and interests of the broad range of individuals and groups who are affected by the ethical conflict and will be harmed by or will benefit from the decision. The challenge in responding to an ethical conflict is choosing among potential options and their underlying values. This frequently involves prioritizing competing values. There are no simple answers to the issue of ranking priorities; however, the organization's mission and value statements may provide guidance when ranking the interests or values of one over another. It has been suggested that because the fundamental purpose of a healthcare organization is quality patient care, the ranking of competing priorities should be as follows: first, patients or the population served; second, clinicians and staff; and third, the organization itself, including its financial stability (see P. H. Werhane, "Business Ethics, Stakeholder Theory, and the Ethics of Healthcare Organizations," *Cambridge Quarterly of Healthcare Ethics,* 2000, 9:169–81). The ranking of these potentially competing priorities and values in this or any order is controversial. Similar to a process of addressing competing moral principles, there is no absolute ranking. Instead, the discussion pushes our reasoning by asking when, if ever, we are justified in not giving patient care first priority (see D. Ozar, J. Berg, P. H. Werhane, and L. Emanual, "Organizational Ethics in Health Care: Toward a Model for Ethical Decision Making by Provider Organizations," *Institute for Ethics National Working Group Report,* American Medical Association, 2001).

A MULTISTEP ETHICAL DECISION-MAKING PROCESS

The following process reflecting procedural justice can help healthcare executives respond to common, yet challenging, organizational ethical conflicts in a planned, systematic manner.

Whether used by an individual or a group, such as your organization's ethics committee, the process can enhance the quality of decisions by helping you clarify ethical conflicts, structure your reasoning, and promote ethical standards of practice.

STEP ONE: CLARIFY THE ETHICAL CONFLICT

What is the specific ethical question or conflict?

You should be able to clearly and succinctly articulate the ethical question that needs to be answered. The parties involved in the process should agree that it is an ethical question or that the question has ethical ramifications. This step is crucial, because if all the parties do not agree on the specific ethical question, reaching agreement on a response will be difficult and even unlikely. In the Memorial Medical Center case outlined above, the situation does raise an ethical conflict between addressing community healthcare needs and functioning as a financially responsible medical center. Does MMC have an ethical obligation to close the clinic to maintain the financial security of the entire medical center, or does it have an ethical obligation to keep the clinic open to provide needed care to the community?

What if the question or conflict is not an ethical question?

If the conflict is not an ethical question, it should be referred to another person or process. For example, if it is a purely legal question, consult with legal counsel. However, many situations may have ramifications in several areas, such as compliance, law, and/or ethics, in which case using the organizational ethics decision-making process would be appropriate for fostering dialogue between the various perspectives.

STEP TWO: IDENTIFY ALL OF THE AFFECTED STAKEHOLDERS AND THEIR VALUES

Who are the individuals or programs affected by the ethical question?

In the MMC example, the ethics issue raises many related concerns, including financial concerns. Therefore, it is appropriate to involve the organization's financial officer in the discussion. Several others ought to participate as well, including community representatives, patients, clinicians, the clinic administrator, representatives from the management team, legal counsel, members of the governing board, and an ethics expert.

What are the values and perspectives of all the affected stakeholders?

Each stakeholder should be given the opportunity to express his or her values-driven perspective. In most cases, the easiest way to do this is to simply ask. For example, Memorial Medical Center may want to have a discussion with some of the potentially affected patients about how they would obtain healthcare services if the clinic no longer operated in their community.

Such a discussion can also be an opportunity to educate community members about the issue: "We know that this clinic is important to you, but it's also a financial drain on our organization. What do you think we should do about this?" Patients and community members won't be able to articulate a financial plan for rescuing the clinic, but such questioning does involve them more in the nature of the problem and allows them to see the organization's perspective while at the same time giving them an opportunity to present theirs. This process should then be repeated with other stakeholders, such as financial officers and physicians.

STEP THREE: UNDERSTAND THE CIRCUMSTANCES SURROUNDING THE ETHICAL CONFLICT

This step requires extensive fact-finding, including why the ethical question has arisen and in what situation and how it is currently addressed in the organization or specific department. You will also need to identify the economic, patient care, legal, and/or community concerns. In the MMC case, the group will need to carefully review many facts related to the ethical conflict: Why is the clinic losing money? What strategies have been employed to balance patient care and financial stability? Why is this particular clinic losing money while others do not? What are the implications to the organization and to the community if the clinic closes? How severe are the financial losses, and what are the specific implications if the losses continue?

STEP FOUR: IDENTIFY THE ETHICAL PERSPECTIVES RELEVANT TO THE CONFLICT

To effectively respond to an ethics question, you must identify relevant ethical concepts. Depending on the particular ethical question, explore the relationship of the ethical question to ethical thinking, including professional codes such as ACHE's *Code of Ethics;* organizational and business ethics literature and position papers; your organization's policies and procedures; and ACHE's *Ethical Policy Statements.* In the MMC example, the group will need to reflect on such concepts as fiduciary relationships as well as communitarian and individualistic ethical perspectives. This step pushes ethical reasoning, exploring the conflict through the lenses of ethical concepts.

STEP FIVE: IDENTIFY DIFFERENT OPTIONS FOR ACTION

What are the possible options for responding to the ethical conflict or question?

In the MMC example, there are obvious options: Close the clinic and encourage patients to seek healthcare at another site, or keep the clinic open, realizing that financial losses may continue. But there are other less obvious approaches as well. MMC may develop and employ new strategies to reduce the financial drain to a more acceptable level while maintaining high-quality care. In discussing various courses of action, be open to many options without prematurely eliminating any option.

Healthcare executives might be quick to say that MMC must close the clinic because it has an obligation to maintain its overall financial security. But it is important to review carefully all of the options and the values driving each one before ruling anything out. MMC's management team may want to consider certain questions: Is MMC for-profit or not-for-profit, and should this affect the decision? Why is so much of the care at the clinic not being reimbursed? What are the Medicaid policies of the state that MMC is in? During this step, you should also consult with colleagues or ethicists to see how similar issues have been addressed at other organizations. Considering all of the issues surrounding the facts can raise additional approaches to resolving the conflict.

What is the ethical reasoning for each option?

Once the different options have been identified, articulate the ethical reasoning that supports each option. In the MMC case, there is an ethical argument for closing the clinic based on the value of preserving MMC's overall financial stability—allowing it to continue to provide quality care to other patients and communities. But there is also an ethical argument for keeping the clinic open based on the value of maintaining a fiduciary relationship to its patients and the community, regardless of the ability to pay.

STEP SIX: SELECT AMONG THE OPTIONS

Have you systematically and quantitatively evaluated each option?

Each option should be carefully assessed regarding its benefits and costs in relationship to the overall mission and value statements of the organization. Costs are not limited to the financial; they can include public relations, employee morale, or consumer service. Also consider the likelihood of the consequences occurring and the degree of uncertainty surrounding each option.

Is the option practical? Does it have a clear ethical foundation?

If an option is impractical, it may need to be passed over. For example, an option may create a significant economic burden. The decision to eliminate a particular option for such reasons needs to occur only after thoughtful review. The option that is selected should not only be practical; it should also be based on clinical and organizational ethical principles and be synergistic with the organization's mission and value statements.

Does one ethical concept or stakeholder value appear to be stronger than the others?

This question relates to the ranking of the options, including various stakeholders' interests and values in response to the specific question. Consider whether one option appears stronger than another. Will infringing on one stakeholder perspective protect or promote another? Is this infringement necessary? In addition, consider how the different options will appear to others and whether you will be able to publicly justify your decision by articulating your ethical reasoning for selecting a particular option. Considering the public ramification of each option at this point is important because once a final decision is made, you will need to openly share it with the stakeholders. As noted earlier, it is in the ranking of the competing values that the controversies occur. In the case of MMC, the preamble to ACHE's *Code of Ethics* can be a helpful resource in weighing the competing values: "The fundamental objectives of the healthcare management profession are to maintain or enhance the overall quality of life, dignity and well-being of every individual needing healthcare service and to create a more equitable, accessible, effective and efficient healthcare system."

STEP SEVEN: SHARE AND IMPLEMENT THE DECISION

Organizational decisions should be publicly disclosed along with the ethical reasons behind them. In the case of MMC, if the organization elects to close the clinic, it is not acceptable to just tack a notice on the door of the clinic announcing that it will be closing. Instead, MMC leaders might consider holding a town hall meeting with the staff of the clinic, patients, and community members, to let them know what actions are planned over the coming months and why. This type of meeting brings the decision-making process out from behind closed doors and promotes better relations with the stakeholders. The different parties will not always agree with the final decision, but they will know that the organization thought through the decision and considered all perspectives before making that decision. In this case, MMC may want to take an even more proactive approach by inviting local media to the town hall meeting or sending a press release to the local paper. Doing so can demonstrate to stakeholders that although it was a painful decision, it is what MMC believes to be the right decision.

Looking for More Ethics Resources?

As more instances of corporate misconduct surface in the media each day, healthcare executives and their organizations may feel the need for ethics resources outside of those available within their immediate organizational setting. To that end, ACHE has developed an Ethics Toolkit, a group of practical resources to help healthcare executives

---

(Continued on following page)

understand how to integrate ethics into their organizations. These tools can support healthcare leaders in the day-to-day practice of exemplary leadership. In addition to the ethical decision-making process outlined in this article, the toolkit provides guidance in understanding and applying ACHE's *Code of Ethics, Ethical Policy Statements*, and *Ethics Self-Assessment* and suggests additional readings and guidelines that can augment decision making. Contents include:

- **Strengthening Ethical Decision Making:** An article that offers strategies senior leaders can use to enhance their ethical awareness and make better ethical decisions
- **Using ACHE's *Code of Ethics*:** An explanation of the history and purpose of the *Code of Ethics* and how it can be used in practical, everyday situations
- **Using ACHE's *Ethical Policy Statements*:** Strategies for applying ACHE's specific policy statements, such as "Decisions Near the End of Life," to your decisions and your organization's policy development
- **Using ACHE's *Ethics Self-Assessment*:** Tips for getting the most out of an ethics self-audit, and how to address potential red flags that you may identify in the process
- **Additional Ethics Resources:** A list of books, magazine and journal articles, periodicals, and Web sites that can provide additional ethics guidance

To access the Ethics Toolkit, go to www.ache.org/see/ethics.

STEP EIGHT: REVIEW THE DECISION TO ENSURE IT ACHIEVED THE DESIRED GOAL

Assessing the outcome of the decision can be a formal or informal process. If MMC elects to close the clinic, a formal assessment option would be to survey all of the patients who were being cared for by that clinic, asking questions such as "Do you have a new healthcare provider?" and "Has the clinic closure caused significant health-related problems for you or your family?" A more informal process would be to select a few representatives of the community and solicit their perception of the effect of the clinic closure. If MMC elects to keep the clinic open, assessment would involve looking at the financial situation periodically to see whether it has improved or at the very least has not gotten worse. If the situation becomes worse, the *facts* of the ethical question have changed, and then the decision may need to be reevaluated.

If it becomes clear that the course of action did not achieve the anticipated outcome, then the organization should reconsider the decision and explore other options based on the current information. On the other hand, if the decision *did* lead to the desired outcome, the organization should evaluate whether the decision can be used to shape responses to other ethical dilemmas. Documenting the case can build an important organizational resource on which to draw in future ethical conflicts.

To foster the efficiency and effectiveness of the decision-making process, healthcare executives should be open to comments from all stakeholders regarding the process.

A CALL TO ACTION

Healthcare executives must address many recurring organizational ethical conflicts such as allocating resources or questions concerning clinical practices. How you respond to these problems will influence your organization's success and quality of care. As a healthcare executive, it is your responsibility to ensure that ethical questions are thoughtfully reviewed prior to any decision. In addition to having clearly established, shared values—including the organization's mission, code of ethics, values statement, and ethical standards of practice—every organization needs an effective ethics infrastructure and process to provide clarification when ethical conflicts arise. Using a deliberative, systematic decision-making process such as the one outlined above can help you promote ethical standards of practice and ensure that ethical conflicts are appropriately addressed.

July/August 2005

ACHE Ethics Committee
Scope and Function

THE *CODE OF ETHICS* is administered by the Ethics Committee, which is appointed by the Board of Governors upon nomination by the Chairman. It is composed of at least nine Fellows of ACHE, each of whom serves a three-year term on a staggered basis, with three members retiring each year. The Ethics Committee shall:

- Review and evaluate annually the *Code of Ethics*, and make any necessary recommendations for updating the *Code*.
- Review and recommend action to the Board of Governors on allegations brought forth regarding breaches of the *Code of Ethics*.
- Develop ethical policy statements to serve as guidelines of ethical conduct for healthcare executives and their professional relationships.
- Prepare an annual report of observations, accomplishments, and recommendations to the Board of Governors, and such other periodic reports as required.

The Ethics Committee invokes the *Code of Ethics* under authority of the ACHE *Bylaws,* Article II, Membership, Section 6, Resignation,

Suspension and Expulsion of Affiliates; Reclassification and Former Affiliate Status, subsection (b), as follows:

Affiliates may be suspended or expelled by action of the Board of Governors as a result of violation of the *Code of Ethics*; nonconformity with the *Bylaws* or *Regulations Governing Admission, Advancement, and Recertification;* conviction of a felony; or conviction of a crime of moral turpitude or a crime relating to the healthcare management profession. No such suspension or expulsion shall be effected without affording a reasonable opportunity for the affiliate to consider the charges and to appear in his or her own defense before the Board of Governors or its designated hearing committee, as outlined in procedures adopted by the Board of Governors.

Selected Healthcare Ethics Bibliography

GENERAL HEALTHCARE ETHICS

American College of Physicians. 1998. "Ethics Manual, 4th ed." *Annals of Internal Medicine* 128 (7): 576–94.

American Hospital Association. 1994. *Values in Conflict: Ethical Issues in Health Care*, 2nd ed. Chicago: American Hospital Association.

Barnett, K., and M. Pittman. 2001. "Doing Good and Doing Well." *Healthcare Forum Journal* 44 (3): 12–19.

Blustein, J., L. Post, and N. Dubler. 2002. *Ethics for Health Care Organizations: Theory, Case Studies, and Tools.* New York: United Hospital Fund of New York.

Boyle, P., E. DuBose, S. Ellingson, D. Guinn, and D. McCurdy. 2001. *Organizational Ethics in Health Care: Principles, Cases, and Practical Solutions.* San Francisco: Jossey-Bass.

Catholic Health Association. 1991. *Corporate Ethics in Healthcare.* St. Louis, MO: CHA.

Chaiken, M., R. Porter, and I. Schick. 2001. "Core Competencies in Ethics." *Journal of Health Administration Education* (Special Issue) 149–57.

Daniels, N., and J. Sabin. 2002. *Setting Limits Fairly: Can We Learn to Share Medical Resources?* New York: Oxford University Press.

Darr, K. 2004. *Ethics in Health Services Management*, 4th ed. Baltimore, MD: Health Professions Press.

Devettere, R. 2000. *Practical Decision Making in Health Care Ethics: Cases and Concepts*, 2nd ed. Washington, DC: Georgetown University Press.

Friedman, E. 2008. "Never Events and Health Care Ethics."[Online article; retrieved 11/2/09.] www. hhnmag. com/hhnmag_app/jsp/articledisplay. jsp?dcrpath=HHNMAG/Article/data/04APR2008/080401H HN_Online_Friedman&domain=HHNMAG.

———. 1996. *The Right Thing: Ten Years of Ethics Columns from the Healthcare Forum Journal.* San Francisco: Jossey-Bass.

Friedman, E., ed. 1992. *Choices and Conflict: Explorations in Health Care Ethics.* Chicago: American Hospital Association.

Grafius, L. 1995. *Ethics for Everyone: A Practical Guide to Interdisciplinary Biomedical Ethics Education.* Chicago: American Hospital Publishing Inc.

Griffith, J. 1993. *The Moral Challenges of Health Care Management.* Chicago: Health Administration Press.

Hall, R. 2000. *An Introduction to Healthcare Organizational Ethics.* New York: Oxford University Press.

Hiller, M. 1986. *Ethics and Health Administration: Ethical Decision Making in Health Management.* Arlington, TX: Association of University Programs in Health Administration.

Hofmann, P., and W. Nelson, eds. 2001. *Managing Ethically: An Executive's Guide*. Chicago: Health Administration Press.

Kuczewski, M., and R. Pinkus. 1999. *An Ethics Casebook for Hospitals: Practical Approaches to Everyday Cases*. Washington, DC: Georgetown University Press.

Nash, L. 1981. "Ethics Without the Sermon." *Harvard Business Review* 59 (6): 79–90.

Nelson, W. 2008. "Rural Health Care Ethics: An Overview." In *Rural Ethics Reader*, edited by C. Klugman, 34–59. Baltimore: The Hopkins Press.

———. 2006. "Defining Ethics." *Healthcare Executive* 21 (4): 38–39.

Nelson, W., and J. Schmidek. 2008. "Rural Healthcare Ethics." In *The Cambridge Textbook of Bioethics*, edited by P. Singer and A. Viens, 289–98. Cambridge, UK: Cambridge University Press.

Paine, L. 1994. "Managing for Organizational Integrity." *Harvard Business Review* 72 (2): 106–18.

Pearson, S., J. Sabin, and E. Emanuel. 2003. *No Margin, No Mission: Health Care Organizations and the Quest for Ethical Excellence*. New York: Oxford University Press.

Perry, F. 2001. *The Tracks We Leave: Ethics in Healthcare Management*. Chicago: Health Administration Press.

Rachels, J. 1982. "Can Ethics Provide Answers?" *Hastings Center Report* 12 (3): 32–40.

Reiser, S. 1994. "The Ethical Life of Health Care Organizations." *Hastings Center Report* 24 (6): 28–35.

Roberts, L., and A. Dyer, eds. 2004. *Ethics in Mental Health*. Washington, DC: American Psychiatric Publishing, Inc.

Singer, P. A., and A. M. Viens, eds. 2008. *The Cambridge Textbook of Bioethics*. Cambridge, UK: Cambridge University Press.

Spencer, E., A. Mills, M. Rorty, and P. Werhane. 2000. *Organization Ethics in Health Care*. New York: Oxford University Press.

Tamborini-Martin, S., and K. Hanley. 1989. "The Importance of Being Ethical." *Health Progress* 70 (5): 24–27, 82.

Tavis, C., and E. Aronson. 2007. *Mistakes Were Made (But Not by Me): Why We Justify Foolish Beliefs, Bad Decisions, and Hurtful Acts*. Orlando, FL: Harcourt, Inc.

Warnock, G. 1993. "The Object of Morality." *Cambridge Quarterly of Healthcare Ethics* 2 (3): 255–58.

Weber, L. J. 2001. *Business Ethics in Healthcare: Beyond Compliance*. Bloomington, IN: Indiana University Press.

Werhane, P. 1990. "The Ethics of Health Care as a Business." *Business and Professional Ethics Journal* 9 (3, 4): 7–20.

Woodstock Theological Center. 1995. *Ethical Considerations in the Business Aspects of Health Care*. Washington, DC: Georgetown University Press.

Worthley, J. 1999. *Organization Ethics in the Compliance Context: A Healthcare Management Challenge*. Chicago: Health Administration Press.

———. 1997. *The Ethics of the Ordinary in Healthcare: Concepts and Cases*. Chicago: Health Administration Press.

ORGANIZATIONAL ETHICS LEADERSHIP

Aroskar, M. 1994. "The Challenge of Ethical Leadership in Nursing." *Journal of Professional Nursing* 10 (5): 270.

Badaracco, J., and R. Ellsworth. 1989. *Leadership and the Quest for Integrity*. Boston: Harvard Business School Press.

Bryant, L. 2005. "Ethical and Legal Duties for Healthcare Boards." *Healthcare Executive* 20 (4): 46–48.

Collins, J. 2001. "Level 5 Leadership: The Triumph of Humility and Fierce Resolve." *Harvard Business Review* 79 (1): 66–76.

Cooper, T. 1998. *The Responsible Administrator: An Approach to Ethics for the Administrative Role*, 4th ed. San Francisco: Jossey-Bass.

Costa, J. 1998. *The Ethical Imperative: Why Moral Leadership Is Good for Business*. Reading, MA: Perseus Books.

Dolan, T. 2004. "A Time for Ethical Leadership: ACHE Affiliates Can Provide the Moral Leadership Our Nation's Healthcare System Needs." *Healthcare Executive* 19 (1): 6–8.

Dye, C. 2000. *Leadership in Healthcare: Values at the Top*. Chicago: Health Administration Press.

Fenner, K., and M. Basford. 1999. "How Can Leaders Ensure Organizational Integrity?" *Trustee* 52 (3): 26–27.

Friedman, E. 2001. "The Butler Did It." *Healthcare Forum Journal* 44 (4): 5–7.

Gini, A. 1997. "Moral Leadership: An Overview." *Journal of Business Ethics* 16 (3): 323–30.

Hofmann, P. 2008. "The Executive's Role in Malpractice Cases." *Healthcare Executive* 23 (3): 58–59.

———. 2008. "The Myth of Promise Keeping." *Healthcare Executive* 23 (5): 48–49.

———. 2008. "Reevaluating Your Ethical Leadership Skills." *Chief Executive Officer* (Spring) 1, 5, 7.

Jennings, B., B. Gray, V. Sharpe, L. Weiss, and A. Fleischman. 2002. "Ethics and Trusteeship for Health Care: Hospital Board Service in Turbulent Times." *Hastings Center Report Special Supplement* 32 (4): S1–S28.

Kashman, S. 2003. "The Kashman Study: Understanding the Processes Healthcare Executives Use to Resolve Ethical

Issues." Fellowship thesis, American College of Healthcare Executives, Chicago.

Lombardi, D. 1997. *Reorganization and Renewal: Strategies for Healthcare Leaders.* Chicago: Health Administration Press.

May, E. 2005. "Recruiting the Right Management Team for Organizational Transparency." *Healthcare Executive* 20 (4): 22–26.

Messick, D., and M. Bazerman. 1996. "Ethical Leadership and the Psychology of Decision Making." *Sloan Management Review* 37 (2): 9–22.

Ritvo, R., J. Ohlsen, and T. Holland. 2004. *Ethical Governance in Health Care.* Chicago: American Hospital Association.

Rosenthal, A., and M. O'Daniel. 2008. "A Survey of the Impact of Disruptive Behavior and Communication Deficits on Patient Safety." *Joint Commission Journal on Quality and Patient Safety* 34 (8): 464–71.

Safty, A. 2003. "Moral Leadership: Beyond Management and Governance." *Harvard International Review* 25 (3): 84–90.

Sanders, L. 2003. "The Ethics Imperative." *Modern Healthcare* 33 (10): 46.

Taylor, C. 2001. "The Buck Stops Here." *Health Progress* 82 (5): 37–47.

Trevino, L., M. Brown, and L. Hartman. 2003. "A Qualitative Investigation of Perceived Executive Ethical Leadership: Perceptions from Inside and Outside the Executive Suite." *Human Relations* 55: 5–37.

Wieck, K., and K. Sutcliffe. 2001. *Managing the Unexpected: Assuring High Performance in an Age of Complexity.* San Francisco: Jossey-Bass.

ORGANIZATIONAL AND MANAGEMENT ETHICS ISSUES

Batts, C. 1998. "Making Ethics an Organizational Priority." *Healthcare Forum Journal* 41 (1): 38–42.

Bischoff, S., K. DeTienne, and B. Quick. 2000. "Effects of Ethical Stress on Employee Burnout and Fatigue: An Empirical Investigation." *Journal of Nursing Administration* 25: 60–62.

Blake, D. 1999. "Organizational Ethics: Creating Structural and Cultural Change in Healthcare Organizations." *The Journal of Clinical Ethics* 10 (3): 187–93.

Blustein, J., L. Post, and N. Dubler. 2002. *Ethics for Health Care Organizations: Theory, Case Studies, and Tools.* New York: United Hospital Fund of New York.

Boyle, P., E. DuBose, S. Ellingson, D. Guinn, and D. McCurdy. 2001. *Organizational Ethics in Health Care: Principles, Cases, and Practical Solutions.* San Francisco: Jossey-Bass.

Bramstedt, K., and P. Schneider. 2005. "Saying 'Good-Bye': Ethical Issues in the Stewardship of Bed Spaces." *The Journal of Clinical Ethics* 16 (2): 170–75.

Brett, A., J. Raymond, D. Saunders, and G. Khushf. 1998. "An Ethics Discussion Series for Hospital Administrators." *HEC Forum* 10 (20).

Buzachero, V., and J. Gilbert. 2007. "Five Attributes of an Ethical Culture." *Hospitals and Health Networks Online,* June 26.

Cassidy, J. 1998. "Calvary Hospital Focuses on Ethics." *Health Progress* 79 (6): 48–50, 52.

Chervenak, F., and L. McCullough. 2004. "An Ethical Framework for Identifying, Preventing, and Managing Conflicts Confronting Leaders of Academic Health Centers." *Academic Medicine* 79 (11): 1056–61.

———. 2003. "Physicians and Hospital Managers as Cofiduciaries of Patients: Rhetoric or Reality?" *Journal of Healthcare Management* 48 (3): 172–79.

Connor, M., D. Duncombe, E. Barclay, S. Bartel, C. Borden, E. Gross, C. Miller, and P. R. Ponte. 2007. "Creating a Fair and Just Culture: One Institution's Path Toward Organizational Change." *Joint Commission Journal on Quality and Patient Safety* 33 (10): 617–24.

Cook, A., and H. Hoas. 2001. "Voices from the Margins: A Context for Developing Bioethics-Related Resources in Rural Areas." *American Journal of Bioethics* 1 (4): W12.

———. 2000. "Bioethics Activities in Rural Hospitals." *Cambridge Quarterly of Healthcare Ethics* 9 (2): 230–38.

———. 2000. "Where the Rubber Hits the Road: Implications for Organizational and Clinical Ethics in Rural Healthcare Settings." *HEC Forum* 12 (4): 331–40.

DeRenzo, E. 2006. "Individuals, Systems, and Professional Behavior." *The Journal of Clinical Ethics* 17 (3): 275–88.

Dwyer, J. 2002. "Babel, Justice, and Democracy: Reflections on a Shortage of Interpreters at a Public Hospital." *Hastings Center Report* 31 (2): 31–36.

Ehlen, K., and G. Sprenger. 1998. "Ethics and Decision Making in Healthcare." *Journal of Healthcare Management* 43 (3): 219–21.

Emanuel, L. 2000. "Ethics and the Structures of Healthcare." *Cambridge Quarterly of Healthcare Ethics* 9 (2): 151–68.

Fox, E., and J. Tulsky. 2005. "Recommendations for the Ethical Conduct of Quality Improvement." *The Journal of Clinical Ethics* 16 (1): 61–71.

Freed, D. 1992. "The Long Distance Administrator." *Health Management Quarterly* 14 (4): 17–20.

French, P. 1979. "The Corporation as a Moral Person." *American Philosophical Quarterly* 3: 207–15.

Giblin, M., and M. Meaney. 1998. "Corporate Compliance Is Not Enough." *Health Progress* 79 (5): 30–31.

Gilbert, J. 2007. *Strengthening Ethical Wisdom: Tools for Transforming Your Health Care Organization.* Chicago: AHA Press.

Goodstein, J., and B. Carney. 1999. "Actively Engaging Organizational Ethics in Healthcare: Four Essential Elements." *The Journal of Clinical Ethics* 10 (3): 224–29.

Goodstein, J., and R. Potter. 1999. "Beyond Financial Incentives: Organizational Ethics and Organizational Integrity." *HEC Forum* 11 (4): 288–92.

Hall, R. 1999. "Confidentiality as an Organizational Ethics Issue." *The Journal of Clinical Ethics* 10 (3): 230–36.

Heller, J. 1999. "Framing Healthcare Compliance in Ethical Terms: A Taxonomy of Moral Choices." *HEC Forum* 11 (4): 345–57.

Hofmann, P. 2009. "The Use and Misuse of Incentives." *Healthcare Executive* 24 (1): 40–42

———. 2008. "Ethical Issues and Disaster Planning." *Healthcare Executive* 23 (1): 40–41.

———. 2007. "Should Hospitals Always Bill for Costs?" *Healthcare Executive* 22 (4): 38–39.

———. 2006. "Evaluating a Management Candidate's Ethical Fitness." *Healthcare Executive* 21 (3): 34–35.

———. 2006. "The Value of an Ethics Audit." *Healthcare Executive* 21 (2): 44–45.

———. 2005. "Confronting Management Incompetence." *Healthcare Executive* 20 (6): 28, 30.

———. 2005. "The High Cost of Being a Moral Chameleon." *Health Progress* 86 (6): 9–10.

———. 2005. "Responsibility for Unsuccessful Promotions." *Healthcare Executive* 20 (1): 32–33.

———. 2004. "Why Good People Behave Badly." *Healthcare Executive* 19 (2): 40–41.

———. 2003. "Revealing Inconvenient Truths." *Healthcare Executive* 18 (5): 56–57.

———. 2002. "Morally Managing Executive Mistakes." *Frontiers of Health Services Management* 18 (3): 3–27.

———. 1998. "Ethics and the CEO (case commentary)." *Hospitals and Health Networks* 72 (2): 32, 34.

———. 1996. "Achieving Ethical Behavior in Healthcare: Rhetoric Still Reigns Over Reality." *Frontiers of Health Services Management* 13 (2): 37–39.

———. 1996. "Hospital Mergers and Acquisitions: A New Catalyst for Examining Organizational Ethics." *Bioethics Forum* 13 (2): 45–48.

Hofmann, P., and B. Jennings. 2005. "Promoting Advance Directives." *Healthcare Executive* 20 (5): 28, 30.

Hofmann, P., and F. Perry, eds. 2005. *Management Mistakes in Healthcare: Identification, Correction, and Prevention.* Cambridge, UK: Cambridge University Press.

Hofmann, P., and J. Schlosser. 2007. "Assessing Your Probability for Organizational Success." *Healthcare Executive* 22 (3): 50–51.

Howe, E. 1999. "Organizational Ethics' Greatest Challenges." *The Journal of Clinical Ethics* 10 (4): 263–70.

Jansen, L. A., and D. P. Sulmasy. 2003. "Bioethics, Conflicts of Interest, and the Limits of Transparency." *Hastings Center Report* 33 (4): 40–43.

Johnson, K., and K. Roebuck-Colgan. 1999. "Organizational Ethics and Sentinel Events: Doing the Right Thing When the Worst Thing Happens." *The Journal of Clinical Ethics* 10: (3) 237–41.

Joint Commission, The. 1998. *Ethical Issues and Patient Rights Across the Continuum of Care*. Oakbrook Terrace, IL: The Joint Commission.

Kalb, P. 1999. "Health Care Fraud and Abuse." *Journal of the American Medical Association* 282 (12): 1163–68.

Kirby, J., C. Simpson, M. McNally, and F. McDonald. 2005. "Innovative Ways to Instantiate Organizational Ethics in Large Healthcare Organizations." *Organizational Ethics: Healthcare, Business, and Policy* 2 (2): 117–23.

Labb, D. 1999. "Defining Appropriate Care: A Matter of Perspective." *Healthcare Executive* 14 (5): 12–16.

Larson, L. 1999. "The Right Thing to Do." *Trustee* 52 (9): 8–12.

Levey, S., and J. Hill. 1986. "Between Survival and Social Responsibility: In Search of an Ethical Balance." *Journal of Health Administration Education* 4 (2): 225–31.

Mack, J. 2004. "Beyond HIPAA: Ethics in the e-Health Arena." *Healthcare Executive* 19 (5): 32–33.

Midgley, M. 1993. "Must Good Causes Compete?" *Cambridge Quarterly of Healthcare Ethics* 2 (2): 131–39.

Mills, A. 2002. "The Healthcare Organization: New Efficiency Endeavors and the Organization Ethics Program." *The Journal of Clinical Ethics* 13 (1): 29–39.

Morrison, E. 2006. *Ethics in Health Administration: A Practical Approach for Decision Makers*. Chicago: Health Forum.

Nelson, W. 2009. "Conflicts of Interest." *Healthcare Executive* 24 (2): 42–44.

———. 2008. "Addressing Organizational Ethics." *Healthcare Executive* 23 (2): 43–46.

———. 2007. "Dealing with Ethical Challenges." *Healthcare Executive* 22 (2): 36–38.

———. 2006. "Must I Maintain Another Person's Promise?" *Healthcare Executive* 21 (1): 34–35.

———. 2005. "An Organizational Ethics Decision-Making Process." *Healthcare Executive* 20 (4): 9–14.

———. 2004. "Addressing Rural Ethics Issues." *Healthcare Executive* 19 (4): 36–37.

Nelson, W., and J. Campfield. 2008. "Marketing Ethics." *Healthcare Executive* 23 (6): 44–45.

———. 2006. "Ethical Implications of Transparency." *Healthcare Executive* 21 (6): 33–34.

Nelson, W., and P. Gardent. 2008. "Ethics and Quality Improvement." *Healthcare Executive* 23 (4): 40–41.

Nelson, W., J. Neily, P. Mills, and W. Weeks. 2008. "Collaboration of Ethics and Patient Safety Programs: Opportunities to Promote Quality." *HEC Forum* 20 (1): 15–27.

Nelson, W., and A. Pomerantz. 1992. "Ethics Issues in Rural Health Care." *Trustee* 45 (8): 14–15.

Nelson, W., W. Weeks, and J. Campfield. 2008. "The Organizational Costs of Ethical Conflicts." *Journal of Healthcare Management* 53 (1): 41–52.

Oak, J. 2005. "Accepting Vendor Gifts." *Healthcare Executive* 20 (4): 32–33.

Olson, R. 1999. "The Postmodern Prescription: An Antidote to Hard Boundaries and Closed Systems in Healthcare Organizations." *The Journal of Clinical Ethics* 10 (3): 178–86.

Ozar, D., J. Berg, P. Werhane, and L. Emanuel. 2001. "Organizational Ethics in Health Care: Toward a Model for Ethical Decision Making by Provider Organizations." *Institute for Ethics National Working Group Report.* Chicago: American Medical Association.

Relman, A. 1994. "Physicians and Business Managers: A Clash of Cultures." *Health Management Quarterly* XVI (3): 11–14.

Ritvo, R., J. Ohlsen, and T. Holland. 2004. *Ethical Governance in Health Care.* Chicago: American Hospital Association.

Rovner, J. 1998. "Organizational Ethics: It's Your Move." *Health System Leader* 5 (1): 4–12.

Rudnick, J. 1995. "Hospital Layoffs: One Facility's Experience with a Work Force Reduction." *Health Progress* 76 (7): 26–29.

Schyve, P. 1996. "Patient Rights and Organization Ethics: The Joint Commission Perspective." *Bioethics Forum* 12 (2): 13–20.

Seely, C., and S. Goldberger. 1999. "Integrated Ethics: Synecdoche in Healthcare." *The Journal of Clinical Ethics* 10 (3): 202–9.

Silva, D., J. Gibson, R. Sibbald, E. Connolly, and P. A. Singer. 2008. "Clinical Ethicists' Perspectives on Organizational Ethics in Health Care Organizations." *Journal of Medical Ethics* 34: 320–3.

Spencer, E., and A. Mills. 1999. "Ethics in Healthcare Organizations." *Healthcare Ethics Committee Forum* 11 (4): 345–57.

Taylor, M. 2003. "Getting in Step with Integrity Pacts." *Modern Healthcare* 33 (47): S12.

Walshe, K., and S. Shortell. 2004. "When Things Go Wrong: How Health Care Organizations Deal with Major Failures." *Health Affairs* 23 (3): 103–11.

Weaver, G., and L. Treviño. 1999. "Compliance and Values Oriented Ethics Programs: Influences on Employees' Attitudes and Behavior." *Business Ethics Quarterly* 9: 315–35.

Weber, L. 1997. "Taking on Organizational Ethics." *Health Progress* 78 (3): 20.

Werhane, P. 2000. "Ethics, Stakeholder Theory, and the Ethics of Healthcare Organizations." *Cambridge Quarterly of Healthcare Ethics* 9 (2): 169–81.

Winkler, E., and R. Gruen. 2005. "First Principles: Substantive Ethics for Healthcare Organizations." *Journal of Healthcare Management* 50 (2): 109–19.

MISSION AND CODE OF ETHICS

American College of Healthcare Executives. 2004. "Code of Ethics." *Annual Report and Reference Guide* 54–55. (Also available at www.ache.org/ABT_ACHE/code.cfm.)

Arbuckle, G. 1999. "Mission and Business: Resolving the Tension." *Health Progress* 80 (5): 22–24, 28.

Bianco, D. 1998. "Considering Conversion?" *Trustee* 51 (10): 16–20.

Brien, A. 1996. "Regulating Virtue: Formulating, Engendering and Enforcing Corporate Ethics Codes." *Business and Professional Ethics Journal* 15 (1): 21–52.

Carlson, G. 1998. "Mission Possible." *Healthcare Executive* 13 (2): 52–53.

Nelson, W., and P. Schurr. 2003. "Affiliates Comment on Code of Ethics." *Healthcare Executive* 18 (6): 54–55.

Rocky Mountain Center for Healthcare Ethics. 1998. *Colorado Code of Ethics for Healthcare.* Denver, CO: Rocky Mountain Center for Healthcare Ethics.

Tavistock Group. 1999. "A Shared Statement of Ethical Principles for Those Who Shape and Give Health Care." *Annals of Internal Medicine* 130 (2): 144–47.

Tuohey, J. 1998. "Covenant Model of Corporate Compliance." *Health Progress* 79 (4): 70–75.

Weil, P., and R. Harmata. 2002. "Rekindling the Flame: Routine Practices That Promote Hospital Community Leadership." *Journal of Healthcare Management* 47 (2): 98–109.

MANAGED CARE

Agich, G., and H. Foster. 2000. "Conflicts of Interest and Management in Managed Care." *Cambridge Quarterly of Healthcare Ethics* 9 (2): 189–204.

Buchanan, A. 1998. "Managed Care: Rationing Without Justice, But Not Unjustly." *Journal of Health Politics, Policy and Law* 23 (4): 617–34.

Council on Ethical and Judicial Affairs. 1995. "Ethical Issues in Managed Care." *Journal of the American Medical Association* 273 (4): 330–35.

Emanuel, E. 2000. "Justice and Managed Care: Four Principles for the Just Allocation of Health Care Resources." *Hastings Center Report* 30 (3): 8–16.

Friedman, L., and G. Savage. 1998. "Can Ethical Management and Managed Care Coexist?" *Health Care Management Review* 23 (2): 56–62.

Gervais, K., R. Priester, D. Vawter, K. Otte, and M. Solberg. 1999. *Ethical Challenges in Managed Care: A Casebook.* Washington, DC: Georgetown University Press.

Greene, J. 1997. "Has Managed Care Lost Its Soul?" *Hospitals and Health Networks* 71 (10): 36–42.

Jacobson, P., and M. Cahill. 2000. "Applying Fiduciary Responsibilities in the Managed Care Context." *American Journal of Law, Medicine and Ethics* 26 (2, 3): 155–73.

Khushf, G. 1999. "The Case for Managed Care." *Journal of Medicine and Philosophy* 24 (5): 415–550.

Morreim, E. 1999. "Assessing Quality of Care: New Twists from Managed Care." *The Journal of Clinical Ethics* 10 (2): 88–99.

———. 1995. *Balancing Act: The New Medical Ethics of Medicine's New Economics.* Washington, DC: Georgetown University Press.

Paris, J., and S. Post. 2000. "Managed Care, Cost Control, and the Common Good." *Cambridge Quarterly of Healthcare Ethics* 9 (2): 182–88.

Pellegrino, E. 1997. "Managed Care at the Bedside: How Do We Look in the Moral Mirror?" *Kennedy Institute of Ethics Journal* 7 (4): 321–30.

Perkel, R. 1996. "Ethics and Managed Care." *Medical Clinics of North America* 80 (2): 263–78.

Randel, L., S. Pearson, J. Sabin, T. Hyams, and E. Emanuel. 2001. "How Managed Care Can Be Ethical." *Health Affairs* 20 (4): 43–56.

Veatch, R. 1997. "Who Should Manage Care?" *Kennedy Institute of Ethics Journal* 7 (4): 391–401.

Veatch, R., and C. Spicer. 1997. "Ethical Challenges in Managed Care." *Kennedy Institute of Ethics Journal* 7 (4).

RESOURCE ALLOCATION AND COST CONTAINMENT

Asch, D., and P. Ubel. 1997. "Rationing by Any Other Name." *New England Journal of Medicine* 336 (23): 1668–71.

Boyle, P., and E. Moskowitz. 1996. "Making Tough Resource Decisions." *Health Progress* 77 (6): 48–53.

Callahan, D. 2000. "Rationing, Equity, and Affordable Care." *Health Progress* 81 (4): 38–41.

Cochran, C., J. Kupersmith, and T. McGovern. 2000. "Justice, Allocation, and Managed Care." *Health Progress* 81 (4): 34–37, 41.

Daniels, N. 1986. "Why Saying No to Patients in the United States Is So Hard." *New England Journal of Medicine* 314 (21): 1380–83.

Emanuel, E. J. 2000. "Justice and Managed Care: Four Principles for the Just Allocation of Health Care Resources." *Hastings Center Report* 30 (3): 8–16.

Grumbach, K., and T. Bodenheimer. 1994. "Painful vs. Painless Cost Control." *Journal of the American Medical Association* 272 (18): 1458–64.

Halter, M. 2004. "When Is It OK to Ration Healthcare?" *Healthcare Executive* 19 (6): 30–31.

Pendola, C. J. 1992. "Administrative Ethics in Health Care Resource Allocation." *Review of Business* 14: 20–22.

Powers, M., and R. Faden. 2000. "Inequalities in Healthcare: Four Generations of Discussion About Justice and Cost-Effectiveness Analysis." *Kennedy Institute of Ethics Journal* 10 (2): 109–27.

Repenshek, M. 2004. "Stewardship and Organizational Ethics: How Can Hospitals and Physicians Balance Scarce Resources with Their Duty to Serve the Poor?" *Health Progress* 85 (3): 31–35, 56.

Ubel, P., and S. Goold. 1997. "Recognizing Bedside Rationing: Clear Cases and Tough Calls." *Annals of Internal Medicine* 125 (1): 74–80.

CLINICAL ETHICS ISSUES

Baily, M., M. Bottrell, J. Lynn, and B. Jennings. 2006. "The Ethics of Using QI Methods to Improve Health Care Quality and Safety." *Hastings Center Report Special Supplement* 36 (4): S1–S39.

Balcerzak, G., and K. Leonhardt. 2008. "Alternative Dispute Resolution in Healthcare: Prescription for Increasing Disclosure and Improving Patient Safety." *Patient Safety and Quality Healthcare* 5 (4): 44–48.

Berger, J., and F. Rosener. 1996. "The Ethics of Practice Guidelines." *Archives of Internal Medicine* 156 (18): 2051–56.

Cook, A., H. Hoas, and K. Guttmannova. 2002. "Ethical Issues Faced by Rural Physicians." *South Dakota Journal of Medicine* 55 (6): 221–4.

DeRenzo, E., P. Panzarella, S. Selinger, and J. Schwartz. 2005. "Emancipation, Capacity, and the Difference Between Law and Ethics." *The Journal of Clinical Ethics* 16 (2): 144–50.

Diekema, D. 2007. "The Armchair Ethicist: It's All About Location." *The Journal of Clinical Ethics* 18 (3): 227–32.

Dubler, N., and C. Liebman. 2004. *Bioethics Mediation: A Guide to Shaping Shared Solutions.* New York: United Hospital Fund of New York.

Glover, J. 2001. "Rural Bioethical Issues of the Elderly: How Do They Differ from Urban Ones?" *Journal of Rural Health* 17 (4): 332–35.

Hilfiker, D. 1984. "Facing Our Mistakes." *New England Journal of Medicine* 310: 118–22.

Hofmann, P. 2009. "Addressing Compassion Fatigue." *Healthcare Executive* 24 (5) 40–42.

———. 2008. "The Executive's Role in Malpractice Cases." *Healthcare Executive* 23 (3): 58–59.

———. 2007. "Ethical Questions at the End of Life." *Healthcare Executive* 22 (1): 37–39.

———. 2006. "Responding to Clinical Mistakes." *Healthcare Executive* 21 (5): 32–33.

———. 2006. "When Patients Make 'Unwise' Decisions." *Hospitals and Health Networks Online* June 13.

———. 2005. "Accountability for Nosocomial Infections." *Healthcare Executive* 20 (3): 48–49.

———. 2001. "Navigating Differences in Patient Values and Preferences." *Healthcare Executive* 16 (2): 58–59.

Hofmann, P., and L. Schneiderman. 2007. "Physicians Should Not Always Pursue a Good 'Clinical' Outcome." *Hastings Center Report* 37 (3): inside back cover.

Howe, E. 2000. "Leaving Luputa: What Doctors Aren't Taught About Informed Consent." *The Journal of Clinical Ethics* 11 (1): 3–13.

Huff, C. 2005. "The Not-So-Simple Truth." *Hospitals and Health Networks* 79 (8): 44–46, 55.

Imhof, S., and B. Kaskie. 2005. "What Do We Owe the Dying? Strategies to Strengthen End-of-Life Care." *Journal of Healthcare Management* 50 (3): 155–68.

Institute of Medicine. 2001. *Crossing the Quality Chasm: A New Health System for the 21st Century*. Washington, DC: National Academies Press.

———. 1999. *To Err Is Human: Building a Safer Health System*. Washington, DC: National Academies Press.

Levinsky, N. 1996. "Social, Institutional, and Economic Barriers to the Exercise of Patients' Rights." *New England Journal of Medicine* 334 (8): 532–34.

Lo, B. 2000. *Resolving Ethical Dilemmas: A Guide for Clinicians*. Philadelphia: Lippincott Williams & Wilkins.

Lynn, J., J. Harrold, and Center to Improve Care of the Dying. 1999. *Handbook for Mortals: Guidance for People Facing Serious Illness*. New York: Oxford University Press.

Martone, M. 2002. "Decision-Making Issues in the Rehabilitation Process." *Hastings Center Report* 31 (2): 36–41.

Mills, A., M. Rorty, and P. Werhane. 2006. "Clinical Ethics and the Managerial Revolution in American Healthcare." *The Journal of Clinical Ethics* 17 (2): 181–90.

Morgenstern, L. 2005. "Proactive Bioethics Screening: A Prelude to Bioethics Consultation." *The Journal of Clinical Ethics* 16 (2): 151–55.

Nelson, W. 2007. "The Ethics of Patient Preferences." *Healthcare Executive* 22 (5): 34, 36–37.

Nelson, W., and P. Gardent. 2008. "Ethics and Quality Improvement." *Healthcare Executive* 23 (4): 40–41.

O'Toole, B. 1998. "Four Ways People Approach Ethics." *Health Progress* 79 (6): 38–41, 43.

Rhodes, R. 1998. "Futility and the Goals of Medicine." *The Journal of Clinical Ethics* 9 (2): 194–205.

Roberts, L., J. Battaglia, and R. Epstein. 1999. "Frontier Ethics: Mental Health Care Needs and Ethical Dilemmas in Rural Communities." *Psychiatric Services* 50 (4): 497–503.

Roberts, L., J. Battaglia, M. Smithpeter, and R. Epstein. 1999. "An Office on Main Street: Health Care Dilemmas in Small Communities." *Hastings Center Report* 29 (4): 28–37.

Rubin, S., and L. Zoloth, eds. 2000. *Margin of Error: The Ethics of Mistakes in the Practice of Medicine.* Hagerstown, MD: University Publishing.

Sharpe, V. 2003. "Promoting Patient Safety: An Ethical Basis for Policy Deliberation." *Hastings Center Report Special Supplement* 33 (5): S1–S20.

Smith, M., and H. Forster. 2000. "Morally Managing Medical Mistakes." *Cambridge Quarterly of Healthcare Ethics* 9 (1): 38–53.

Solovy, A. 1999. "The Price of Dignity." *Hospitals and Health Networks* 73 (3): 30.

Stewart, C. 2005. "Making Decisions About Neonatal Life Support." *Healthcare Executive* 20 (2): 42–43.

Wendler, D., and S. Shah. 2006. "How Can Medical Training and Informed Consent Be Reconciled with Volume-Outcome Data?" *The Journal of Clinical Ethics* 17 (2): 149–57.

Woolf, S. 1999. "The Need for Perspective in Evidence-Based Medicine." *Journal of the American Medical Association* 282 (24): 2358–65.

Wu, A. W., T. A. Cavanaugh, S. J. McPhee, B. Lo, and G. P. Micco. 1997. "To Tell the Truth: Ethical and Practical Issues in Disclosing Medical Mistakes to Patients." *Journal of General Internal Medicine* 12: 770–75.

ETHICS COMMITTEES, PROGRAMS, AND CONSULTATION

American Society for Bioethics and Humanities. 1998. "Core Competencies for Healthcare Ethics Consultation." Glenview, IL: ASBH.

Aroskar, M. 2006. "Healthcare Organizations as Moral Communities." *The Journal of Clinical Ethics* 17 (3): 255–56.

Aulisio, M., R. Arnold, and S. Youngner. 2000. "Health Care Ethics Consultation: Nature, Goals, and Competencies." *Annals of Internal Medicine* 133 (1): 59–69.

Bacchetta, M., and J. Finns. 1997. "The Economics of Clinical Ethics Programs: A Quantitative Justification." *Cambridge Quarterly* 6: 451–60.

Blake, D. C. 2000. "Reinventing the Healthcare Ethics Committee." *HEC Forum* 12 (1): 8–32.

Bushy, A., and J. Rauh. 1991. "Implementing an Ethics Committee in Rural Institutions." *Journal of Nursing Administration* 21 (12): 18–25.

Craig, J. M., and T. May. 2006. "Evaluating the Outcomes of Ethics Consultation." *The Journal of Clinical Ethics* 17 (2): 168–80.

Crigger, B. 1995. "Negotiating the Moral Order: Paradoxes of Ethics Consultation." *Kennedy Institute of Ethics Journal* 5 (2): 89–112.

Dowdy, M., C. Robertson, and J. A. Bander. 1998. "A Study of Proactive Ethics Consultation for Critically and Terminally Ill Patients with Extended Lengths of Stay." *Critical Care Medicine* 26 (2): 252–59.

Dubler, N., and C. Liebman. 2004. *Bioethics Mediation: A Guide to Shaping Shared Solutions.* New York: United Hospital Fund.

Foglia, M., and R. Pearlman. 2006. "Integrating Clinical and Organizational Ethics: A Systems Perspective Can Provide an Antidote to the Silo Problem in Clinical Ethics Consultations." *Health Progress* 87 (2): 31–35.

Gordon, E., and A. Hamric. 2006. "The Courage to Stand Up: The Cultural Politics of Nurses' Access to Ethics Consultation." *The Journal of Clinical Ethics* 17 (3): 231–54.

Harding, J. 1994. "The Role of Organizational Ethics Committees." *Physician Executive* 20 (2): 19–24.

Hirsch, N. 1999. "All in the Family—Siblings but Not Twins: The Relationship of Clinical and Organizational Ethics Analysis." *The Journal of Clinical Ethics* 10 (3): 187–93.

Hofmann, P. 2001. "Improving Ethics Committee Effectiveness." *Healthcare Executive* 16 (1): 58–59.

Kelly, S., P. Marshall, L. Sanders, T. Raffin, and B. Koenig. 1997. "Understanding the Practice of Ethics Consultation: Results of an Ethnographic Multi-Site Study." *The Journal of Clinical Ethics* 8 (2): 136–49.

Lawry, T. 1999. "Ethicists Have Gone Digital." *Health Progress* 80 (5): 10–11.

Mayle, K. 2006. "Nurses and Ethics Consultation: Growing Beyond a Rock and a Hard Place." *The Journal of Clinical Ethics* 17 (3): 257–59.

McCullough, L. 2005. "Practicing Preventive Ethics—The Keys to Avoiding Ethical Conflicts in Health Care." *Physician Executive* 31 (2): 18–21.

———. 1998. "Preventive Ethics, Managed Practice, and the Hospital Ethics Committee as a Resource for Physician Executives." *HEC Forum* 10 (2): 136–51.

McGee, G. 2001. "A National Study of Ethics Committees." *American Journal of Bioethics* 1 (4): 60–64.

Myser, C., P. Donehower, and C. Frank. 1999. "Making the Most of Disequilibrium: Bridging the Gap Between Clinical and Organizational Ethics in a Newly Merged Healthcare Organization." *The Journal of Clinical Ethics* 10 (3): 194–201.

Nelson, W. 2008. "Addressing Organizational Ethics." *Healthcare Executive* 23 (2): 43, 46.

———. 2007. "Ethics Programs in Small Rural Hospitals." *Healthcare Executive* 22 (6): 30, 32–33.

Nelson, W., J. Neily, P. Mills, and W. Weeks. 2008. "Collaboration of Ethics and Patient Safety Programs: Opportunities to Promote Quality." *HEC Forum* 20 (1): 15–27.

Nelson, W., and G. Wlody. 1999. "The Evolving Role of Ethics Advisory Committees in VHA." *Healthcare Ethics Committee Forum* 9 (2): 129–46.

Niemira, D. 1988. "Grassroots Grappling: Ethics Committees at Rural Hospitals." *Annals of Internal Medicine* 109 (12): 981.

Post, L., J. Blustein, and N. Dubler. 2006. *Handbook for Health Care Ethics Committees.* Baltimore: Johns Hopkins University Press.

Potter, R. 1999. "On Our Way to Integrated Bioethics: Clinical/Organizational/Communal." *The Journal of Clinical Ethics* 10 (2): 171–77.

———. 1996. "From Clinical Ethics to Organizational Ethics: The Second Stage of the Evolution of Bioethics." *Bioethics Forum* 12 (2): 3–12.

Renz, D., and W. Eddy. 1996. "Organizations, Ethics, and Health Care: Building an Ethics Infrastructure for a New Era." *Bioethics Forum* 12 (2): 29–39.

Rueping, J., and D. Dugan. 2000. "A Next Generation Ethics

Program in Progress." *HEC Forum* 12 (1): 49–56.

Sabin, J., and D. Cochran. 2007. "From the Field: Confronting Trade-Offs in Health Care: Harvard Pilgrim Health Care's Organizational Ethics Program." *Health Affairs* 26 (4): 1129–34.

Savage, T. 2006. "Physician-Nurse Relationships and Their Effect on Ethical Nursing Practice." *The Journal of Clinical Ethics* 17 (3): 260–65.

Schneiderman, L., T. Gilmer, and H. Teetzel. 2000. "Impact of Ethics Consultations in the Intensive Care Setting: A Randomized Controlled Trial." *Critical Care Medicine* 28 (12): 3920–24.

Scofield, G. 1993. "Ethics Consultation: The Least Dangerous Profession?" *Cambridge Quarterly of Healthcare Ethics* 2 (4): 417–26.

Spencer, E. 1997. "A New Role for Institutional Ethics Committees: Organizational Ethics." *The Journal of Clinical Ethics* 8 (4): 372–76.

HEALTHCARE ETHICS JOURNALS

Cambridge Quarterly of Healthcare Ethics
Cambridge University Press
journals.cambridge.org/action/login

Hastings Center Report
Hastings Center
www.thehastingscenter.org/Publications/HCR/Default
.aspx

HEC Forum
  Kluwer Academic Publishers
  www.springerlink.com/content/102899/

Journal of Business Ethics
  Kluwer Academic Publishers
  www.springer.com/philosophy/ethics/journal/10551

The Journal of Clinical Ethics
  University Publishing Group
  www.clinicalethics.com/

Journal of Law, Medicine & Ethics
  American Society of Law, Medicine & Ethics
  www.aslme.org/pub/jlme/index.php

Journal of Medical Ethics
  BMJ Publishing Group
  jme.bmj.com/

Kennedy Institute of Ethics Journal
  Johns Hopkins University Press
  www.press.jhu.edu/journals/kennedy_institute_of_ethics
  _journal/

SELECTED HEALTHCARE ETHICS–RELATED WEBSITE RESOURCES

American College of Healthcare Executives
www.ache.org

American Journal of Bioethics
www.bioethics.net

American Medical Association Ethics Group
www.ama-assn.org/ama/pub/physician-resources/medical-
    ethics.shtml

American Society for Bioethics and Humanities
www.asbh.org

American Society of Law, Medicine, & Ethics
www.aslme.org

Center for Bioethics, University of Pennsylvania
www.med.upenn.edu/bioethics

Hastings Center
www.thehastingscenter.org

National Center for Ethics in Health Care
www.va.gov/vhaethics

President's Council on Bioethics
www.bioethics.gov

About the Editors

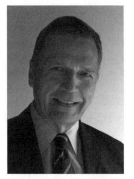

William A. Nelson, MDiv, PhD, is director of Rural Ethics Initiatives and an associate professor of community and family medicine at Dartmouth Medical School and the Dartmouth Institute for Health Policy and Clinical Practice. He also is an adjunct associate professor of public administration at New York University's Robert Wagner Graduate School of Public Service. Previously, he was at the Department of Veterans Affairs' National Center for Ethics in Health Care, which he co-founded. He is the recipient of the United States Congressional Excalibur Award for Public Service, a W. K. Kellogg National Leadership Fellow, and, recently, a National Rural Health Association Leadership Fellow. He received the Department of Veterans Affairs' Under Secretary for Health's highest honor, the Exemplary Service Award. Dr. Nelson received an Honorary Doctorate of Humane Letters from Elmhurst College. He has published extensively in peer-reviewed journals. Dr. Nelson is the principal investigator of several federal- and state-funded research studies fostering an evidence-based approach to ethics and the link between ethics and quality. He is the editor of *Handbook for Rural Health Care: A Practical*

Guide for Professionals, a Dartmouth-based 2009 e-book. In addition to being coeditor of *Managing Ethically: An Executive's Guide,* published in 2001 by Health Administration Press, he is a regular contributor to *Healthcare Executive*'s "Healthcare Management Ethics" column, a consultant to ACHE's Ethics Committee, and a faculty member for ACHE's annual ethics seminar.

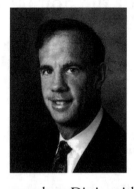

Paul B. Hofmann, DrPH, FACHE, is president of the Hofmann Healthcare Group in Moraga, California. He has been the executive vice president and chief operating officer of the Alta Bates Corporation, a diversified nonprofit healthcare system in northern California; executive director of Emory University Hospital in Atlanta; and director of Stanford University Hospital and Clinics in Palo Alto. He has also served as Distinguished Visiting Scholar at Stanford University's Center for Biomedical Ethics. Dr. Hofmann is a past member of ACHE's Leadership Advisory Committee, and he coordinates the annual ethics conference for ACHE. In addition to being coeditor of *Managing Ethically: An Executive's Guide,* published in 2001 by Health Administration Press, he is coeditor of *Management Mistakes in Healthcare: Identification, Correction and Prevention,* published in 2005 by Cambridge University Press. Dr. Hofmann currently serves on the American Hospital Association McKesson Quest for Quality Prize Committee, The Joint Commission's International Standards Subcommittee, and the board of MedShare International. He is the board chairman of San Francisco–based Operation Access. In 2009, he received the American Hospital Association's Award of Honor for his central role in shaping the field's understanding of healthcare ethics. An author of over 150 publications, Dr. Hofmann has held faculty appointments at Harvard, UCLA, Stanford, Emory, Seton Hall, and the University of California. He earned his undergraduate, master's, and doctor of public health degrees from the University of California.

About the Contributors

Sue G. Brody is president and CEO of Bayfront Health System, headquartered in St. Petersburg, Florida.

Richard Cohan, FACHE, CHC, CCEP, is system director of integrity and compliance and chief privacy officer at Providence Health and Services headquartered in Renton, Washington.

Michael G. Daigneault, Esq., is President of the Ethics Resource Center, a Washington, DC, not-for-profit organization whose vision is an ethical world.

Cedric K. Dark, MD, MPH, is founder and executive editor of policyprescriptions.org, a site dedicated to evidence-based health policy. He is chief resident at the George Washington University Department of Emergency Medicine in Washington, DC.

Benn J. Greenspan, PhD, FACHE, is the MHA program director at the University of Illinois–Chicago School of Public Health. He retired from healthcare delivery after more than 13 years as the CEO of the Sinai Health System of Chicago.

John R. Griffith, FACHE, is the Andrew Pattullo Collegiate Professor, University of Michigan–Ann Arbor, School of Public Health.

John M. Haas, PhD, STL, is president of the National Catholic Bioethics Center in Philadelphia, Pennsylvania.

Gordon C. Hunt, Jr., MD, MBA, is chief medical officer of Sutter Health in Sacramento, California.

John G. King, FACHE, is president of John G. King Associates in Scottsdale, Arizona.

Gloria G. Mayer, RN, EdD, FAAN, is president and CEO of the Institute for Healthcare Advancement in La Habra, California.

Elizabeth S. McGrady, PhD, FACHE, is an assistant professor and program director of the MBA Health Services Management program at the University of Dallas in Irving, Texas. Dr. McGrady has worked in the healthcare field for over 30 years as a clinician, program manager, executive, educator, and consultant.

E. Haavi Morreim, PhD, is professor of bioethics in the College of Medicine, University of Tennessee–Memphis. She has published and lectured extensively on the legal and ethical implications of medicine's changing economics.

Frankie Perry, FACHE(R), serves on the faculty of the Masters of Public Health Program at the University of New Mexico. She is the author of *The Tracks We Leave: Ethics in Healthcare Management*, published by Health Administration Press, and co-author with Paul Hofmann of *Management Mistakes in Healthcare: Identification, Correction, and Prevention*, published by Cambridge University Press. She teaches "Management Mistakes, Ethical Dilemmas, and Lessons Learned," an online seminar offered by ACHE

William D. Petasnick, FACHE, is president and CEO of Froedtert & Community Health in Milwaukee, Wisconsin, and immediate past chairman of the board of trustees of the American Hospital Association.

Edward Petry, PhD, is vice president of the Ethical Leadership Group: A Global Compliance Company.

Michael Villaire, MSLM, is director, Programs and Operations, of the nonprofit Institute for Healthcare Advancement (IHA) in La Habra, California. He directs several IHA initiatives in health literacy, including a continuing education conference and a rewrite/redesign service, available at its website, www.iha4health.org